C000061131

A CENTURY OF ARTERIAL HYPERTENSION

1896-1996

This publication was made possible by a grant
from KNOLL BASF Pharma

A CENTURY OF ARTERIAL HYPERTENSION

1896-1996

Edited by

Nicolas Postel-Vinay

In collaboration with

The International Society of Hypertension

Translated by

Richard Edelstein and Christopher Coffin

JOHN WILEY & SONS / IMOTHEP

Chichester • New York • Brisbane • Toronto • Singapore • Chantilly

Copyright © 1996 by   John Wiley & Sons Ltd,
                         Baffins Lane, Chichester,
                         West Sussex PO19 1UD, England

                         National   01243 779777
                         Telephone   (+44) (1243) 779777
                         e-mail (for orders and customer service enquiries): cs-books@wiley.co.uk
                         Visit our Home Page on   http://www.wiley.co.uk
                                       or   http://www.wiley.com

All Rights Reserved. No part of this book may be reproduced, stored in a retrieval
system, or transmitted, in any form or by any means, electronic, mechanical, photocopying,
recording or otherwise, except under the terms of the Copyright Designs and Patents Act
1988 or under the terms of a licence issued by the Copyright Licensing Agency,
90 Tottenham Court Road, London, UK W1P 9HE, without the permission in writing of the
publisher.

This book was originally published in French under the title:
IMPRESSIONS ARTERIELLES
100 ans d'hypertension 1896 – 1996
ISBN 2-224-02425-8
Copyright © 1996 by   Editions Imothep Médecine-Sciences
                         19, avenue Duquesne
                         75007 Paris, France
                         Telephone (+33)(1) 47 05 84 38

Other Wiley Editorial Offices

John Wiley & Sons Inc., 605 Third Avenue,
New York, NY 10158-0012, USA

Jacaranda Wiley Ltd., 33 Park Road, Milton,
Queensland 4064, Australia

John Wiley & Sons (Canada) Ltd. 22 Worcester Road,
Rexdale, Ontario M9W 1L1, Canada

John Wiley & Sons (Asia) Pte Ltd, 2 Clementi Loop #02-01,
Jin Xing Distripark, Singapore 0512

Wiley Europe (sarl), 14 rue Saint-Laurent
60500 Chantilly, France

British Library Cataloguing in Publication Data

A Catalogue for this book is available from the British Library

ISBN 0 471 96788 2

Printed and bound in Great Britain by Bookcraft (Bath) Ltd, Midsomer Norton, Somerset

Editorial Committee

Michel Beaufils (*Hôpital Tenon, Paris*)
Pierre Corvol (*Collège de France, Paris*)
Frederick Fairhead *(Paris)*
Jacques Guédon (*Hôpital Foch, Suresnes*)
Pavel Hamet *(Hôtel-Dieu, Montreal)*
William Kannel (*Boston University, Framingham*)
Thierry Lang (*Inserm U258, Paris*)
Jean-Michel Mallion (*CHU Grenoble*)
Giuseppe Mancia *(Università degli Studi di Milano, Milan)*
Anne-Marie Moulin (*Inserm U158, Paris*)
Eoin O'Brien *(Beaumont Hospital, Dublin)*
Pierre-François Plouin (*Hôpital Broussais, Paris*)
Nicolas Postel-Vinay (*Inserm U158, Paris*)
Bernard Waeber (*CHU Vaudois, Lausanne*)
Faiez Zannad (*CHU Nancy*)

Acknowledgements

We wish to acknowledge the contributions of the following people whose advice and assistance have been invaluable and whose contributions in reviewing texts, providing original documents and researching historical facts have made this book possible

Kikuo Arakawa, Gilles Chatellier, Jean Deleuze, Edward Freis,
Xavier Jeunemaître, Stevo Julius,
Joël Ménard, Catherine Vincent, Alberto Zanchetti

Nelly Haskett, Bernadette Molitor, Yveline Postel-Vinay,
Marie-France Ruscoe, Bernard Wergens

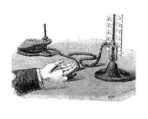

TABLE OF CONTENTS

Preface 1

Foreword

To reflect on a century of hypertension is to understand the emergence and evolution of a new manner of scientific thinking. This book is not a list of dates, but an attempt to understand how the scientific and cultural past has shaped the present. 5

Chapter 1 — Measuring blood pressure

From animals to man: A brief review of early instrumentation and the context in which it was conceived. 9

From measurement to understanding: The methods used and the results obtained. 19

Chapter 2 — Recognising hypertension

The essential contribution of life-insurance companies to the discovery of risk: The view that the invention of the sphygmomanometer led to the discovery of a new disease is too simplistic. The concept of vascular risk began to emerge before the measurement of blood pressure and was the result of a statistical approach. 31

The Framingham enquiry or epidemiology as a research tool: After the Second World War, epidemiology established the idea of multifactorial diseases and the health authorities took over from the private insurance companies. 49

Chapter 3 — Understanding hypertension

Too many questions and an unclassifiable entity: The history of the physiology of hypertension is not linear. Our current understanding derives from the gradual merging of knowledge acquired from many different sources. 59

The discovery of the renin-angiotensin system: The accumulation of two hundred years of medical knowledge by a succession of different approaches: anatomico-clinical first, then experimental, and finally biological. 67

Pheochromocytoma and the concept of surgically curable hypertension: Newly identified clinical syndromes gradually led to the understanding of a cause of secondary hypertension. Surgery played a significant role in this understanding. 79

Conn and aldosteronism: With remarkable perceptiveness, Conn elucidated the endocrinology of blood pressure regulation on the basis of a single clinical case. 87

Chapter 4 — Treating hypertension

The four periods of antihypertensive treatment: During the four periods of antihypertensive treatment, the underlying concepts, the means used and the aims of treatment were perpetually changing. 91

An assorted catalogue of treatments: radiotherapy, electrotherapy, pyrotherapy, surgery and pharmacology: Extraordinarily diverse methods were used in an attempt to lower blood pressure. Many empirical, ineffective, fantastic or dangerous techniques were tried before arriving at the era of modern antihypertensive drugs. 101

Chapter 5 — The question of norms

The fallacy of the dividing line between the normal and the pathological: Potain and Riva-Rocci at the turn of the century, insurance companies between the two world wars, then the World Health Organisation and learned societies after the Second World War all tried to define "normal" blood pressure. General agreement could not be reached and today we recognise that there is no single clear-cut dividing line, but a series of recommendations — all arbitrary. 133

Chapter 6 — Social pressures

Migration and nutrition: hypertension divided between genetics and the environment: Hypertension does not affect all ethnic groups and social classes equally. Blood pressure is subject to the laws of genetics and is influenced by environmental factors. The study of migrating populations and nutritional factors revealed that blood pressure was related to socio-cultural factors that are difficult to interpret.   145

Society under pressure: stress, inequalities and economic pressures: Since blood pressure is related to a subject's emotivity, "stress" and a "modern lifestyle" were accused as far back as the 1920s of being responsible for hypertension. Modern epidemiology has tempered this concept but has not ruled it out completely. Today the treatment of hypertensive individuals has acquired a sociological dimension, in particular because of its financial implications.   155

Chapter 7 — Yesterday's sufferers and today's patients

Towards the disappearance of symptoms: Medical records from the early 20th century, clearly reveal that hypertension was "treated" when it produced symptoms. Today the physician's aim is to intervene before symptoms become apparent, by interpreting the results of tests statistically. Imaging techniques have taken on an important prognostic dimension.   167

Chapter 8 — The genetics of hypertension

Hypertensive families have been reported since 1925. In just over half a century we have progressed from simple epidemiological observation of a hereditary trait to a molecular genetic understanding of the phenomena involved.   181

Epilogue   189

Milestones   191

Biographies   197

Index of names   207

Source of illustrations   213

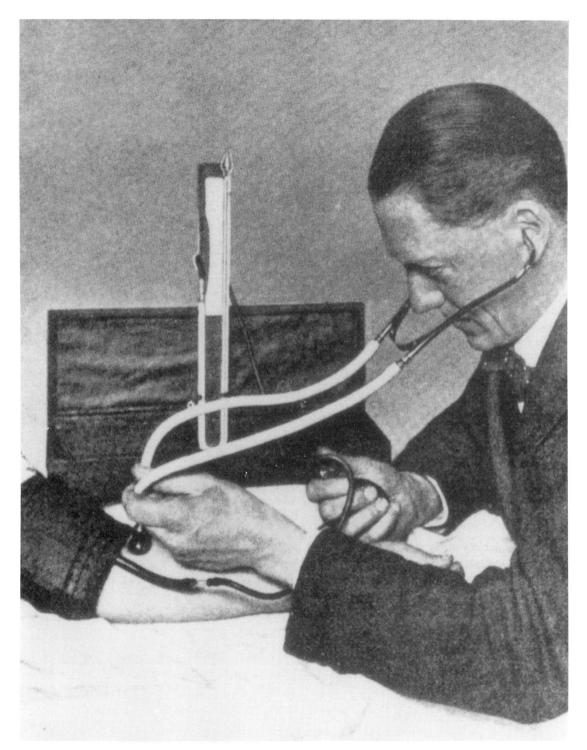

Timeless ?

Riva-Rocci's inflatable cuff combined with Korotkoff's auscultatory method are still in use today. In this photograph, the doctor's hairstyle and dress have aged more quickly than the method he is using. Will it ever become obsolete ?

PREFACE

The International Society of Hypertension is proud and happy to associate with this publication celebrating the "Century of Hypertension". In any field of science and clinical activity, an anniversary should serve to reflect on past accomplishments, present status as well as future orientations.

By a fortunate initiative of the "Société Française d'Hypertension Artérielle", under the historical guidance of Doctor Nicolas Postel-Vinay, "Year 1" of hypertension was established in 1896. Very appropriately, the documentation of Riva-Rocci's sphygmomanometer in the *Gazzetta Medica di Torino* - December 17, 1896, was a major starting point in the development of hypertension as a research and clinical activity.

From the early appreciation of hypertension as a clinical entity to the grasp of its epidemiological relevance, from early treatment attempts to the therapeutic success of the present and tomorrow's discoveries of the molecular genetic foundations of the disease, this book walks the reader from the pioneering past to the fascinating future in our field.

The International Society of Hypertension has declared 1996 as the year of the 100th Anniversary of Hypertension, and, indeed, a Century of Achievements.

Professor Kikuo Arakawa

President
International Society
of Hypertension

Professor Pavel Hamet

Secretary
International Society
of Hypertension

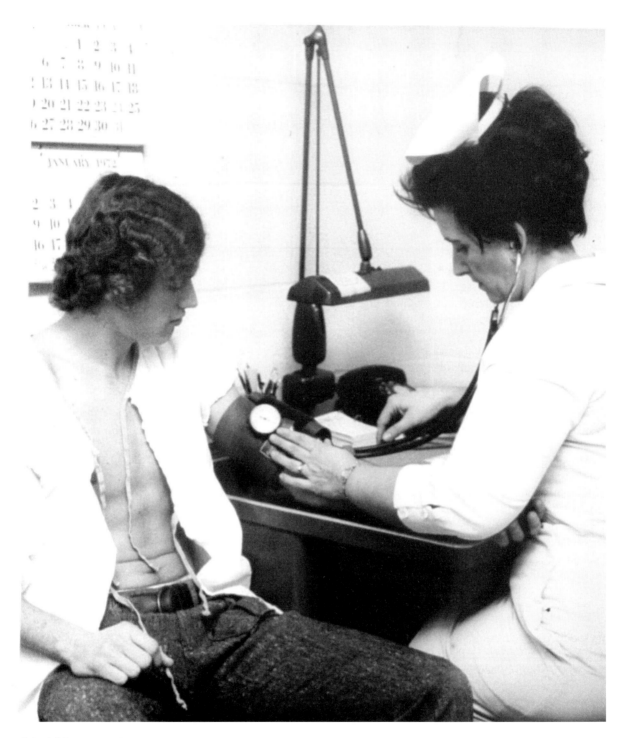

Arterial hypertension: the culprit

After World War II, the Framingham study confirmed what insurance companies had been proclaiming: high blood pressure is a major risk factor for vascular disease. The methodological recommendation was to have the patient seated.

Commemorations of all sorts are becoming increasingly frequent. It is as though, in the changing fortunes of our Western societies, the lives and work of our predecessors symbolise a stable cultural value.

Medicine is becoming increasingly technological and the traditional doctor-patient relationship is changing. In this context, it would appear opportune to look back and reflect on the achievements of our chosen field, not simply to recollect the facts for the sake of scholars of history but, more broadly, to comprehend where medicine stands today and where tomorrow's developments might lead us.

Curiously, hypertension, despite its prevalence, has been the subject of very few historical analyses. There are some accounts of the history of blood pressure measurement but little attention has been devoted to the evolution of the concept of risk and and of hypertension itself.

Hypertension as a clinical concept is exactly 100 years old and on this occasion the French Society of Hypertension wished to pay a tribute to Scipione Riva-Rocci whose invention of the inflatable cuff in 1896 provided us with a simple and reliable method for the clinical measurement of blood pressure, without which our field would not be where it is today.

The Society also wished to encourage the publication of a book which highlights the achievements of the past 100 years and reflects on the evolution of ideas surrounding hypertension.

The International Society of Hypertension took an interest in the project and judged that the book warranted wider readership than was possible in its original French edition. This is now possible with the publication of the English-language edition. We are honoured by the interest that the International Society has expressed for the project, and grateful for its support.

We would like to thank all those who have joined us in commemorating 'A CENTURY OF ARTERIAL HYPERTENSION'. Our thanks go to all the contributors and particularly to the editor, Dr. Nicolas Postel-Vinay. We would also like to acknowledge the support of KNOLL BASF Pharma, whose generous support has made this book possible.

Jean-Michel Mallion
President of the French Society of Hypertension

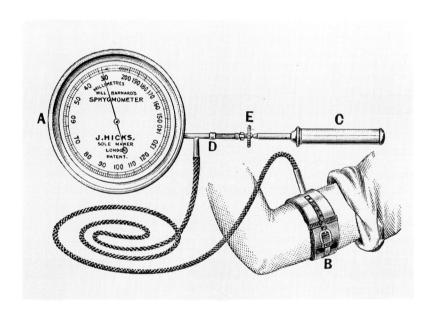

FOREWORD

The history of hypertension presented in this book is a panorama of the evolution of ideas and views on arterial hypertension. Our aim is to lead the reader through the past one hundred years of the history of hypertension and to show how this history contributed to the emergence of modern medicine.

As an entity, hypertension grew as one scientific building block was added to another, but its overall configuration was not the work of science alone. Fields as diverse as ethics, economics, sociology and philosophy have all had an increasing influence as they evolved in their own right over the past hundred years.

It was exactly one hundred years ago, in 1896, that hypertension earned its rightful place as an integral part of medicine, if we consider the reference point to be the development of the inflatable cuff by Riva-Rocci — a milestone for the measurement of blood pressure in man.

Some might argue that the reference point is situated earlier, starting with the first physiological studies of blood pressure measurement in animals in 1773. Others will claim that the real starting point was the emerging concept of high blood pressure as a risk factor in the first decade of the twentieth century.

To publish a book reflecting on the development of this concept is tempting from several viewpoints. First, the historical, because to the best of our knowledge no such work on the subject has ever been published.

Sociological, because vascular risk factors have an enormous social impact. And finally, epistemological, because the conceptions of arterial hypertension create a fascinating relationship between the body and medicine, between humans and numbers. With hypertension, hyperbole is never far away. Who would venture to guess the number of hypertensive individuals in the world today? Looking back on his career, a major actor on the hypertensive scene described the awe he experienced in the face of *"the enormous sums of money, the swarms of technicians, the ubiquitous committees and task-forces, prestige importantly based on money, the occasional overt fraud, the avalanche of reading matter and the big-time politics"* associated with hypertension.[1]

At the turn of the century, physicians concentrated on severe, symptomatic hypertension. Today they are looking at some 15% of the population in industrialised nations. Hypertension is *"the Triumph of Medicine"* to quote Dr. Knock in a famous French satirical play by Jules Romains[2]. Surely any physician diagnosing mild essential hypertension in one of his patients would not dispute the memorable words of Jules Romains: *"To fall ill is an outdated concept which is untenable in the face of modern science. Health is but a word, with which our vocabulary could readily dispense. As for myself, I know only of people who are more or less afflicted with a greater or less number of ailments which follow a more or less rapid course. Naturally if you tell them that they are well, they are all too inclined to believe you — but you are deceiving them"*. They are hypertensive, one would wish to add!

Hypertension is an entity defined by numbers rather than by signs and symptoms. But it also calls for a verbal description, not because the quantitative approach is deficient, but because it can be complemented and enriched by a historical, sociological, epistemological and economic analysis.

The centenary of the invention by Riva-Rocci of an effective method for measuring blood pressure at the bedside provides us with an opportunity to reflect upon how the measurement of blood pressure has become a routine act, deeply entrenched in the scientific culture of all practising physicians. Certain pathophysiological studies have suggested that high blood pressure is related to the "stress" associated with modern life in industrialised countries. This view portrays hypertension as a disease of civilisation, or of "the American way of life" as stated in 1931[3]. Twenty years later, epidemiologists moderated this view and considered that hypertension was the reflection of an ageing civilisation which, having conquered infectious diseases and infant mortality, could now turn its attention to degenerative disorders. While it might be true to say that hypertension is a consequence of modern medicine, it is equally true that it is one of its inventions. Discovered as a result of the commercial pursuits

1. Irvine Page. *Hypertension research. A memoir.* 1920-1960. Pergamon Press, N.Y. 1988.

2. Jules Romains. *Knock ou le Triomphe de la médecine.* 1923.

3. David Riesman. High blood pressure and longevity. *JAMA* 1931. 96; 14 : 1105-1111.

of life insurance companies, defined arbitrarily and situated beyond the usual anatomico-clinical boundaries, hypertension acquired its current status of a major public health problem just after the end of the Second World War.

Arterial hypertension, a concept rather than a disease, is a fascinating phenomenon to observe because its existence, its history, and the issues at stake are one of the best reflections of what contemporary medicine is all about. The discovery of antibiotics is vivid in people's minds as a major historic event, and many works have dealt with its history. In contrast, the fight against hypertension has not inspired historians and sociologist to the same degree, no doubt owing to the lack of a spectacular lightning victory, as was the case with bacterial infections.

And yet, to look back over a hundred years of hypertension is to observe how medicine has evolved over the past century. The realisation that hypertensive patients needed to be cared for constituted a turning point in the evolution of contemporary medicine. This book aims to examine the impact of the past on the present and to answer the question: "How did we get to where we are?"

Nicolas Postel-Vinay

1
MEASURING BLOOD PRESSURE

From animals to man

"The action of the heart has such a profound effect on blood flow that we believe physiologists should be focusing their attention on new research concerning the force of this organ. We know that age, sex, temperament, idiosyncrasy, sleep and wakefulness, exercise, rest, a state of health or disease and the passions all affect the force of the heart to a greater or lesser degree. We recognise the influence of these modifying agents, but does their existence prohibit further work to determine the limits of this force? We do not believe so".

J.L.M. Poiseuille
*Recherches sur la force du coeur aortique
(Research on the force of the aortic heart)*
Doctoral thesis, Paris 1828.

The earliest measurements of blood pressure by Hales in 1773 and Poiseuille in 1828, were performed in mares and dogs. An artery had to be severed to connect the manometer, so on each occasion the animal paid the price of its life to satisfy man's scientific curiosity. Such experiments did not appear feasible in humans, and yet in 1856, Faivre a surgeon from Lyons, connected the femoral or humeral artery of patients undergoing amputation to a mercury manometer (similar to the Ludwig kymograph). He recorded "mean pressures" of 115 to 120 mmHg. But such experiments remain marginal in the history of human arterial pressure [1].

Clearly, another approach — an indirect approach — was needed. The working principle of an indirect approach emerged from the development of a technique designed to study the pulse: the sphygmograph. It was in 1834 that Hérisson devised a new instrument to *"provide a visual reflection of the action of the arteries"*. The sphygmometer was a simple and ingenious instrument which simply applied a column of mercury to an artery of the forearm (radial artery). Unlike Poiseuille's haemodynamometer, the procedure was non-invasive, consisting simply of external application over the artery rather than surgical insertion into the artery. Fitted with an elastic membrane applied to the patient's wrist, Hérisson's sphygmometer (built by the engineer Paul Gernier) aimed to

1. We have been unable to find the original reference. Vaschide and Lahy refer to these invasive measurements in humans but they do not mention the investigators' names: *"The study of blood pressure by inserting cannulae into arteries cannot be used in humans, though it is true that some surgeons have taken advantage of the opportunity offered by amputations to apply the method. Few results are available and they do not satisfy the needs of either clinical medicine or of psychophysiology"*. (Vaschide and Lahy in: *Archives Générales de Médecine*. La technique de la mesure de la pression sanguine (Technique for measuring blood pressure) 1902, pp. 480-501).

replace the classical ancestral palpation of the pulse which 18th century physicians had refined to a degree now long forgotten (except in Chinese medicine). With the apparatus, the pulse was no longer felt, but seen. The observer saw the vertical oscillations of a column of mercury, "*a fleeting and difficult phenomenon to analyse*" in the words of Marey. The procedure needed to be improved. This task was taken on by the German school of physiology which invented a new scientific language: graphic recording [2].

THE GRAPHIC METHOD: A QUEST FOR OBJECTIVITY

With the advent of the graphic method, the sphygmometer became the sphygmograph. A small metal stylet scraping across smoke-blackened paper translated the pulsations of the radial artery into graphic waves. This technical innovation was intended to supplant the finger or the eye of a human observer with an objective and reproducible method. The sphygmograph was the first medical device to eliminate the need for the human senses, touch and sight, in this case.

Vierodt, who conceived the sphygmograph, suggested that the counter-pressure required to suppress the pulse beats could provide an indirect assessment of the blood pressure [3]. The principle behind this idea was of great importance, even if at the time it was not technically feasible. Marey, himself the inventor of one of the most accurate sphygmographs (1860), recognised that this method was unable to provide reliable values for blood pressure [4]. The sphygmograph was, nonetheless, an important tool in cardiology, useful for studying cardiac rhythm and certain forms of valvular disease. Sphygmography became increasingly popular with more enlightened physicians at the end of the 19th century and, an important fact, it was used in the second half of the 19th century by physicians working for life insurance companies to assess the degree of atherosclerosis in applicants. The sphygmograph was thus the first investigational tool in cardiovascular medicine (Laënnec's stethoscope had been used since the early 19th century but was really part of the clinical examination). And so, for the first time in cardiovascular medicine, an apparatus left the physiologist's laboratory to become an integral part of the practitioner's armamentarium. This event did not, of course, concern the majority of physicians. For one thing, interpreting the tracings was difficult and, for another, the apparatus was expensive [5].

In pioneering the use of a non-invasive investigational technique, the sphygmograph encouraged other physicians to attempt to develop a similar instrument capable of measuring blood pressure in humans. Victor Basch in Vienna devised such an instrument. In 1880 he described a sphygmomanometer consisting of an elastic pouch connected to a manometer. The pouch was applied to the wrist with increasing pressure until the pulsations of the radial artery disappeared.

2. For more on the history of graphic recording, see the study by Francois Dagonet entitled *Etienne Jules Marey.* 1987. Hazan, Paris.

3. Karl Vierodt: *Die Lehre von Arterienpuls* (A treatise on the pulse). 1855. Braunschweig F. Vieweg.

4. E.J. Marey. *La Circulation du sang à l'état physiologique et dans les maladies* (Blood circulation in health and disease).1881. Paris. "*In any valid study of blood pressure, we must abandon the use of the sphygmograph to obtain absolute values and we must be content to gain but an indirect indication of this pressure from observing the shape of the pulse waves*".

5. The sphygmograph was of use essentially for qualitative evaluation of the pulse based on the shape of the curve obtained. The latter changed according to the rigidity of the artery, heart rate and the presence of valvular heart disease. Many different types of sphygmograph were devised and something like fifty versions made their appearance in Europe during the second half of the nineteenth century. Marey's sphygmograph was probably one of the more reliable ones. Dudgeon's had the advantage of being simple to use and was popular in England. Weighing only 120 grams, it could easily be transported in a leather case.

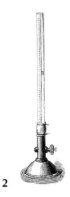

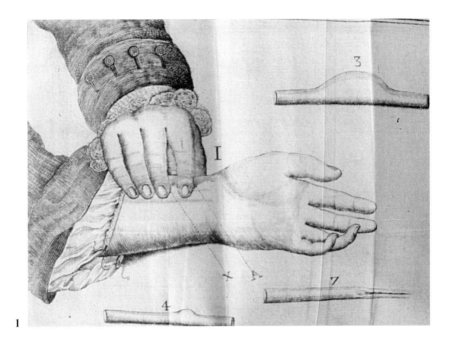

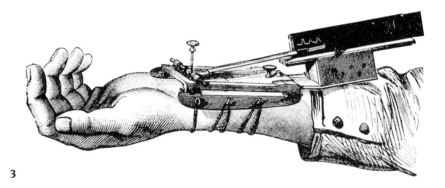

The sphygmometer and the sphygmograph: early attempts to study blood flow in humans with the aid of an apparatus.

Palpation of the pulse had been performed as far back as Hippocrates and remained very much in vogue in the 17th and 18th centuries *(figure 1)*. The technique was revolutionised in the 19th century with the invention of the sphygmometer *(Hérisson, 1834)*. The first model consisted simply of a column of mercury applied to the radial artery *(figure 2)* but it was perfected by a number of scientists who devised many different models. Marey's sphygmograph *(1860)* incorporated an accurate system of graphic recording *(figure 3)*, enabling objective study of the movements of the radial pulse. The sphygmograph thus overcame the problem of the human examiner's subjective evaluation and paved the way for the use of reproducible investigational techniques.

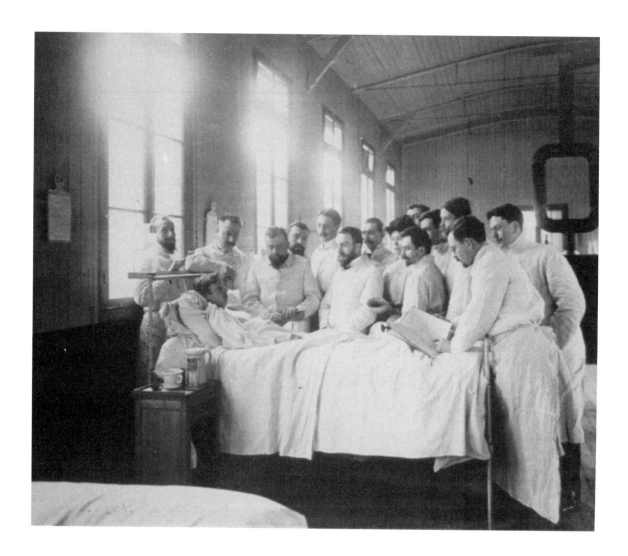

Measuring blood pressure at the turn of the century: a ceremonial

In the years 1880-1900, Basch and Potain introduced the measurement of blood pressure during hospital ward rounds. It had not yet become a routine procedure. This photograph, taken at the Hôpital de La Charité around 1910, shows Henri Vaquez measuring the systolic blood pressure of a patient with a Potain sphygmomanometer. Performed by the department head in person, the procedure was difficult... and photogenic.

The blood pressure recordings performed in this way were actually fairly accurate [6]. In France, the clinician Potain, enthused and inspired by Basch's invention, went on to build a new instrument. With the advent of these two instruments, the great adventure of simple and non-invasive measurement of blood pressure in humans was about to begin. Basch and Potain were the first two physicians to introduce sphygmomanometry into the hospital setting.

6. Victor Basch. *Ueber die Messung des Blutdrucks am Menschen*. (On the measurement of blood pressure in man) *Zt Klin Med* 1880; 2: 79-96.

1896: A TURNING POINT FOR THE ACCURACY OF BLOOD PRESSURE MEASUREMENT

Following in the footsteps of Basch and Potain, numerous physicians, physiologists, engineers and manufacturers embarked upon the adventure of trying to improve the indirect measurement of blood pressure. Many models were built but few were ever used in the clinic. The year 1896 marked a turning point. The Italian physician Riva-Rocci fitted the sphygmomanometer with an inflatable cuff, thus heralding the modern era of blood pressure recording. He presented his discovery at the Italian Congress of Internal Medicine and his paper was published the same year [7].

Riva-Rocci's invention was quickly adopted throughout Italy, Great Britain and the United States but encountered some difficulty in crossing the Alps into France, no doubt because of the hegemony of Potain's sphygomanometer. Riva-Rocci presented his invention to the French medical community in an article published in *La Presse Médicale* (November 1899), shortly after the journal had published another article recommending the use of Potain's sphygmomanometer, which was technically inferior to Riva-Rocci's apparatus. Here is what Riva-Rocci had to say: *"In issue 33 of La Presse Médicale, Doctor Millian stresses the very great clinical importance of measuring blood pressure and he even cites some indirect clinical signs derived from the inspection and the palpation of the heart and pulse. But the author also rightly emphasises the shortcomings of the method and its sources of error. Doctor Millian therefore rightly recommends the use of Potain's sphygmomanometer as the best way of measuring the blood pressure clinically. This sphygmomanometer is almost identical to that of Basch. I myself began my studies using this apparatus which is quite ingenious. But, as many investigators have remarked, it is too often subjected to causes of error and the values it gives differ when used by different observers [...]. In trying to improve on Professor Potain's apparatus, I came up with a new device which appears to me to be simple, easy to apply and provides accurate readings which are constant from one examiner to another. I presented my new sphygmomanometer to the Italian Congress of Internal Medicine back in 1896. The manufacturers tell me that they are supplying doctors in several foreign countries, especially Germany, England and America.*

7. Riva-Rocci S. Un nuovo sfigmomanometro. (A new sphygmomanometer) *Gazzetta Medica di Torino.* 1896; 47: 981-1001.

On reading Dr. Millian's article I realised that it had gone unnoticed in France. I have therefore given a brief description of my apparatus and I hope that my honourable French colleagues, who have played such a dominant role in the study of arterial pressure, will give me their opinion after having tested it".

The rest is history. The utility of the inflatable cuff (later enlarged for better accuracy) to measure blood pressure by exerting a counter-pressure sufficient to close the artery was clear. The technique really came into its own with the introduction of the auscultatory method described in 1905 by the Russian surgeon Nicolaï Korotkoff. During the preparation of his doctoral thesis in Saint Petersburg on the subject of the diagnosis and treatment of arterial and venous trauma, Korotkoff noticed that the pulse wave produced an audible bruit on auscultation of the artery compressed by a cuff.

Nicolaï Korotkoff (1874-1920) presented his discovery in 1905 to the Imperial Academy of Medicine. His presentation was published in Russian. *"On the basis of his observations, the investigator* (Korotkoff) *came to the conclusion that a totally compressed artery produces no sound whatsoever under normal conditions. Given this principle, the investigator proposes the auscultatory method to determine blood pressure in humans. The cuff of Riva-Rocci is placed on the middle third of the upper arm; the pressure within the cuff is quickly raised up to complete cessation of circulation below the cuff. Then, letting the mercury of the manometer fall, one listens to the artery just below the cuff with a children's stethoscope. At first no sounds are heard. With the falling of the mercury in the manometer down to a certain height, the first short tones appear; their appearance indicates the passage of part of the pulse wave under the cuff. It follows that the manometric figure at which the first tone appears corresponds to the maximal pressure. With the further fall of the mercury in the manometer one hears the systolic compression murmurs, which pass again into tones (second). Finally, all sounds disappear. The time of cession of sounds indicates the free passage of the pulse wave; in other words, at the moment of the disappearance of the sounds the minimal blood pressure within the artery predominates over the pressure in the cuff. It follows that the manometric figures at this time correspond to the minimal blood pressure. Experiments in animals have given positive results. The first sounds become audible before the pulse can be felt, as the latter requires the major part of the blood to flow through the artery"* [8].

In 1919, Vaquez et Laubry signed a contract with the manufacturer Spengler for the commercial production of a sphygmotensiophone, which is still used today. This instrument was simple and inexpensive and provided the means for measuring blood pressure in large numbers

8. Nicolaï Korotkoff. To the question of methods of determining the blood pressure (from the clinic of Professor C.P. Federoof). *Reports of the Imperial Military Academy.* 1905; 11: 365-367.

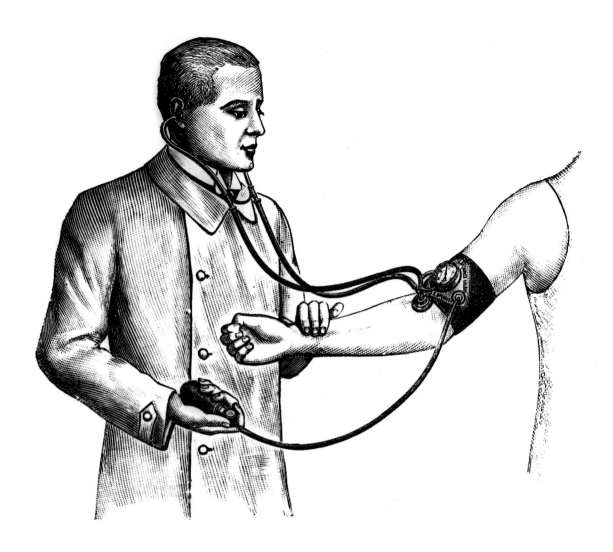

The auscultatory method: towards the measurement of diastolic blood pressure

The apparatuses designed by Basch and Potain provided only the values of the systolic blood pressure. In 1905 the Russian surgeon Nicolaï Korotkoff described an auscultatory method thereby paving the way for indirect measurement of the diastolic blood pressure. The combination of the cuff invented by Riva-Rocci and auscultation of arterial bruits led to the design of the sphygmotensiophone. The model developed by Vaquez and Laubry with the manufacturer Spengler is still used today. In 1917, Fischer introduced the measurement of blood pressure as one of the tests required by life insurance companies. He recommended that the diastolic blood pressure be taken into account and in 1921 he convened a blood pressure committee which, the following year, made recommendations concerning the relevance of the diastolic pressure.

of patients. It is clear from articles in the French medical press of
the time that Potain's apparatus continued to be widely used even
though it had been made obsolete by Riva-Rocci's invention. In the
early twentieth century, measuring devices thus became an integral
part of the study of hypertension. However this labile physiological
parameter was still of obscure significance and its complex regulatory
mechanisms remained unknown.

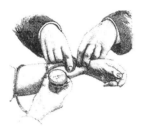

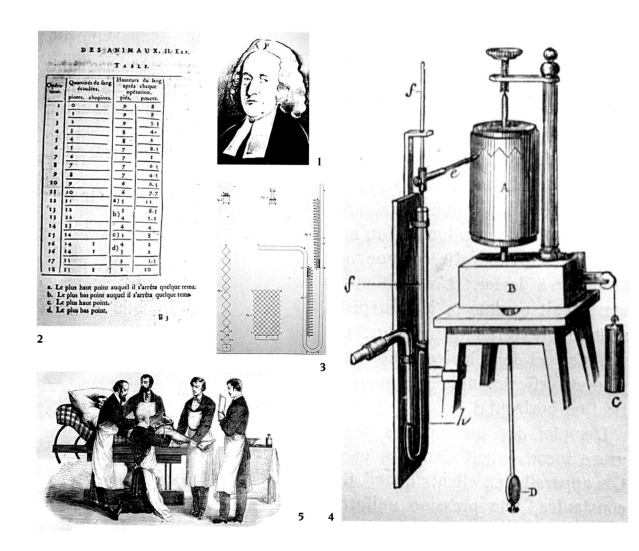

Invasive measurements of blood pressure

The first experimental measurement of blood pressure in animals was performed by Stephen Hales using a simple copper cannula *(figure 1)*. Hales immediately noted the oscillating nature of the blood pressure as reflected in the table taken from his work *"An account of some hydraulic and hydrostatical experiments made on the blood and blood vessels of animals"*, published in 1733 and translated into French in 1744 *(figure 2)*. The first instrument designed specifically for measuring blood pressure was Poiseuille's "haemodynamometer" (1838) *(figure 3)*, which was succeeded by Ludwig's "kymograph" (1846). This instrument had the advantage of being fitted with a graphic recording system *(figure 4)*.

This type of apparatus was used in animals in physiology laboratories but it was also exceptionally used by daring surgeons during amputations of the lower extremity in humans *(figure 5)*. From 1733 until 1880 these experimental measures were performed with no clinical consideration in mind.

From measurement to understanding

" As an animal body consists not only of a wonderful texture of solid parts, but also of a large proportion of fluids, which are continually circulating and flowing thro' an inimitable embroidery of blood-vessels, and other inconceivably minute canals; and as the healthy state of an animal principally consists, in the maintaining of a due equilibrium between those solids and fluids; it has ever since the important discovery of the circulation of the blood, been looked upon as a matter well worth the inquiring into, to find the force and velocity with which these fluids are impelled; as a likely means to give a considerable insight into the animal oeconomy".

Stephen Hales
London 1733

It was in the 18th century that Stephen Hales broke ground into the investigation of the relationship between measurement and human health. In these very early days of measurement of blood pressure, he noted great variability in the readings obtained [1].

1. Hales S. *An account of some hydraulic and hydrostatical experiments made on the blood and blood vessels of animals.* 1733. London.

After connecting a curved copper tube to the crural artery of a mare, he remarked that the column of blood rose and fell with each beat of the heart. He studied this phenomenon on some 25 consecutive occasions in the same mare and observed the variability of the pressure depending on the movements of the animal, its pulse, its respiration and its degree of exhaustion or fright.

Variability was noted very early on in the history of measurement of blood pressure and quickly gave rise to a multitude of investigations [2]. From the second half of the 19th century, physiologists described the infinite subtleties of what was then known as the "sphygmomanometric technique". Entire volumes were devoted to this new science, one of the most famous being Marey's *Blood circulation in health and disease* which was published in 1881, was 750 pages long and included 360 figures.

2. For details on the history of the introduction of measurement into the biological sciences, see M.D. Grmek. *La Première Révolution Biologique* (The First Biological Revolution) 1990. Payot, Paris.

Marey's work was really the start of a new chapter, that of the variation and variability of blood pressure, that is an understanding of blood pressure based essentially on the evolution of measurement techniques rather than on clinical, epidemiological or pathophysiological observations. For over a century, and up to the present day, much has been written about blood pressure levels observed in different circumstances using a variety of different apparatuses. Since the time of the first manometers used in animals (Poiseuille 1818), to the use of Basch's sphygmomanometer (1880) and up to modern-day instruments, all derived from the concepts of Riva-Rocci and Korotkoff, there has been a long list of innovations (but also technical failures) which have refined our understanding of blood pressure. Today, the evaluation of a patient with hypertension has evolved from taking static readings (simply recording the systolic and diastolic pressures) to a dynamic approach based on a computer analysis of measurements derived from 24-hour recordings.

It is not our intention to summarise the history of measurement techniques. There have been many detailed articles dealing with the subject [3]. It may be useful however to reflect on the relationship between the history of measurement and the evolution of our knowledge of hypertension. To describe an apparatus is one thing, to understand the context in which it was used is another. A sphygmomanometer does not provide the same information in the hands of a physiologist, an insurance agent, an epidemiologist or a clinician. Because blood pressure is such a physiologically and pathologically variable parameter, measuring it raises major problems of methodology (which apparatus? what recommendations for use?), of diagnosis (what are normal values?) and of prognosis (how to interpret?).

The medical literature abounds with questions — and even quarrels — about methodology. Each investigator invented a "personal" method of measurement and pre-occupation with technical aspects sometimes turned attention away from the real questions raised by the recognition of hypertension as a vascular risk factor (in contrast, articles on therapy during this period were often insufficiently explicit about the methodology of measurement).

A number of authors believed they had devised more effective instruments than Riva-Rocci's manometer combined with the auscultatory method of Korotkoff. The wave-like nature of blood pressure suggested the idea of using recording devices (such as Boulitte's recording oscillometer first proposed at the turn of the century). Pachon conceived his oscillometer which remained in use for a long time. Paillard invented a rather singular "cervical water manometer". The apparatus consisted of the inner tube of a bicycle tyre placed around the neck and connected to a water manometer. By means of this procedure, the author was able to measure the jugular venous pressure using Valsalva's manoeuver [4].

3. See in particular: O'Brien E., Fitzgerald D. The history of blood pressure measurement. *Journal of Human Hypertension* 1994; 8: 73-84. It is noteworthy however that articles on the history of blood pressure measurement deal essentially with the technical aspects. There is no complete treatise on the epistemological aspects of measurement and a book on the intellectual context of the research done by Hales, Marey, Ludwig, Potain or Riva-Rocci would be most welcome.

4. The author went one step further and also proposed a "water sphygmomanometer to measure quite small differences in the blood pressure". The instrument was 2.72 m high!
H. Paillard. Sphygmomanomètre à eau (A water sphygmomanometer). *Le Journal Médical Français*; February 1933, p. 50.

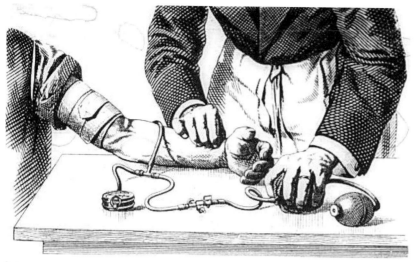

2

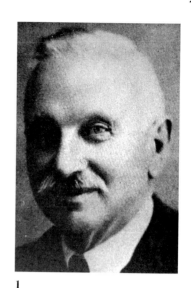

1

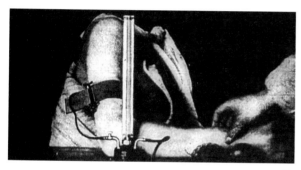

3

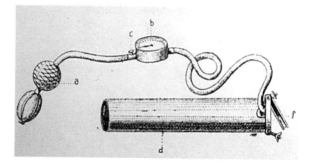

4

1896 : Riva-Rocci's cuff

After making his presentation to the Italian Congress of Internal Medicine, the Italian physician Scipione Riva-Rocci (1863-1937) (*figure 1*) published his "nuovo sfigmomanometro" in the *Gazetta Medica di Torino* of December 17, 1896.

Riva-Rocci's sphygmomanometer was based on the principle of Basch and Potain. The innovation was the possibility of cutting off the humeral circulation by means of a *"band which could be gradually tightened by means of a tourniquet" (figures 2 and 3)*. Riva-Rocci then perfected his technique by conceiving a cuff consisting of a *"chamber, like the inner tube of a bicycle tyre"* surrounded by an *"inextensible cuff" (figure 4)*.

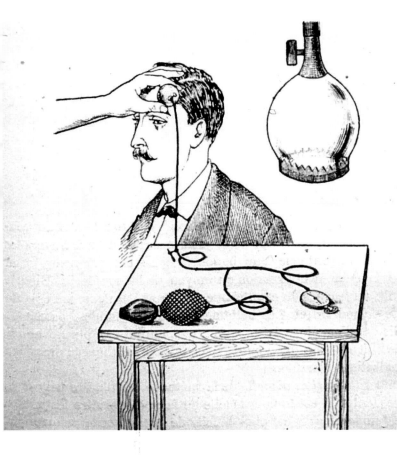

Anecdotal devices for measuring blood pressure

The indirect measurement of blood pressure was attempted by methods others than that of Riva-Rocci. Most of them were quickly forgotten but they do reflect, anecdotally, the inventiveness and imagination of certain physicians.

In 1895, the Italian Mosso conceived a device which totalised blood pressure at the extremities of the four fingers (*bottom right*) (see footnote 7).

In 1920, a device for measuring blood pressure at the level of the temporal artery (*top*) was proposed in an article which appeared in the *Archives du Coeur, des Vaisseaux et du Sang* (1920, pp. 445-446). According to this procedure, the pressure in the temporal artery was 3 cmHg in the normal subject.

In 1933, readers of the *Journal Médical Français* (volume XXII, p. 48) discovered "a cervical water manometer" (*bottom left*) (see footnote 4).

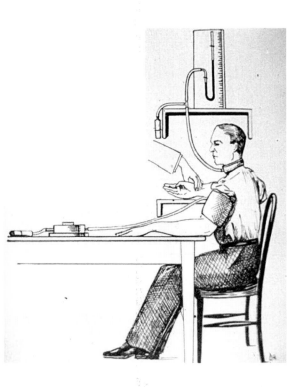

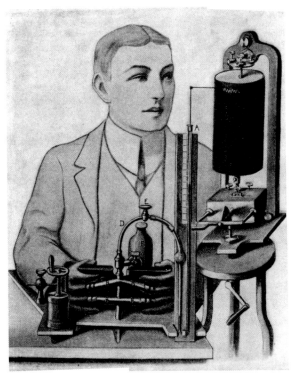

As was to be the case for therapeutic procedures, the first twenty years witnessed a whole host of innovative measuring devices, none of which stood the test of time. Essentially, it can be said that there were no decisive technical inventions between 1900 and 1960. It was not until the 1960s that new methods for the continuous ambulatory measurement of blood pressure shed new light on the study of hypertension.

In 1960, M. Sokolow and his co-workers used a semi-automatic instrument to measure blood pressure in ambulatory patients. In 1962, Hinman, Engel and Bickford [5] used a portable non-invasive system of blood pressure measurement. In 1966, a direct intra-arterial system (the so-called Oxford system) for continuous recording was tested by Bevan, Honour and Stott [6]. More recently, it became possible to record blood pressure continuously by a non-invasive method at the level of the finger. This method accurately reflects the variations, but above all the short-term variability of arterial pressure. These instruments were inspired by the earlier inventions of Mosso and Gaertner who had measured blood pressure in the fingers as far back as the end of the nineenth century [7].

Today, the development of new instruments has been largely fashioned by the progress in electronics which has made modern machines smaller, lighter, more accurate and more reliable. The saga of blood pressure measurement continues with its usual technological and scientific aspects. But today there is also an unprecedented commercial thrust with the prospect of expanding the market beyond doctors and nurses to the immense market of hypertensive patients themselves, who have become the direct targets for major advertising campaigns.

FROM EMOTIONS TO RECOMMENDATIONS

For over a century it has been known that the measurement of blood pressure could be biased by the emotivity of the subject. The well-known "white coat effect", about which so much has been written, is an old story. So old in fact, that as far back as the classical period, physicians palpating the pulse recognised what they called the tachycardia of emotional patients [8]. Looking back, we realise how observant these early investigators were and how relevant their observations remain. Even today, we still find it difficult to overcome this source of bias. Riva-Rocci said it all one hundred years ago when he wrote: *"When the patient has been placed in what we believe to be the best position possible (in usual cases, the patient is sitting on his bed), complete rest and absolute calm are indispensable because even the slightest emotion can cause an appreciable disturbance in*

5. Hinman A.T., Engel B.T., Bickford A.F. Portable blood pressure recorder. Accuracy and preliminary use in the evaluation of intradaily variations in pressure. *Am Heart J* 1962; 63: 663-668.
Kain H.K., Hinman A.T., Sokolow M. Arterial blood pressure measurements with a portable recorder in hypertensive patients. I. Variability and correlation with casual pressure. *Circulation* 1964; 30: 882-892.

6. Bevan A.T., Honour A.J., Stott F. Direct arterial pressure recording in unrestricted man. *Clin Sci* 1969; 36: 329-344.
Bevan A.T., Honour A.J., Stott F. Portable apparatus for the continuous record of intra-arterial pressure. *Clin Sci* 1969; 36: 329.

7. Mosso conceived an apparatus which totalised the blood pressure at the extremity of the four fingers. Mosso. A sphygmomanometer to measure blood pressure in man. *Italian Arch of Biology* 1895, volume XXIII, p. 176. Similarly, Gaertner invented "a pneumatic ring" which was placed on the second phalanx of the finger. G. Gaertner. Ueber einer neuen Blut-druckmesser (tonometer) (On a new apparatus for measuring blood pressure). *Wiener medicinische Wochenschrift* 1899. n°30, pp. 1412-1417.

8. This form of tachycardia induced by the presence of the physician was the object of a historical commentary by Björn Lemmer in a recent letter to the *American Journal of Hypertension* (White coat hypertension: described more than 250 years ago. B. Lemmer. *Am. J. Hypertension.* 1995; 8: 437-438). However, in his reply to the same journal, Thomas Pickering points out that these observations do not prove a rise in blood pressure since the "white coat hypertension phenomenon" is not accompanied by tachycardia.

the level of blood pressure" [9]. Subsequently, a long list of authors, amongst which Potain (1902) [10] and Janeway (1904) [11], drew attention to the variability of blood pressure under the influence of factors such as surgery, smoking or anxiety [12]. At the turn of the century, these observations justified the use of rest as part of the treatment of high blood pressure. But rest was also a confounding factor in many therapeutic studies which claimed to demonstrate the effect of a variety of other anti-hypertensive therapies.

Remarkably, it was not long before precise recommendations for the measurement of blood pressure were made. In an article published in 1912, Gallavardin and Haour advocated waiting five minutes to avoid errors related to the initial hypertension. Gallavardin wrote: *"The apprehensive, impatient or excessively impressionable patient may experience a momentary rise in blood pressure. One must take great care to reassure the patient before taking his blood pressure and above all, several successive measurements should be made"*. He went on to say *"It is an important rule not to continue taking a history during measurement of blood pressure and to wait patiently for the value of the residual systolic pressure [...]. A simple question or a movement by the patient often suffices to determine a re-increase of 10 to 15 mmHg when the drop in blood pressure is very marked"*.

Other authors went even further. Deadborn in 1916 warned that *"it is only by repeating measurements every minute or every two minutes for half an hour on several successive days and by ensuring that one has eliminated all the other known causes of accidental hypertension that one can be sure of having an accurate base for measurement"* [13]. But *"Such a wealth of precautions does indeed appear to be excessive"*, replied Gallavardin.

The advent of portable instruments in recent decades has made it possible to clarify the effects of emotion, anxiety, pain or pleasure which can trigger substantial, unpredictable and sometimes lasting increases in blood pressure. Tests have been devised based on psycho-sensorial stimulation such as mental calculation, mirrors, colour tests or prolonged exposure to unpleasant stimuli such as noise. Studies on "white coat hypertension" have been performed in this context. The rise in blood pressure is concomitant with the arrival of the doctor and reaches a maximum within one to four minutes, then usually disappears after thirty minutes. The reaction is less intense when the blood pressure is taken by a nurse, and self-measurement at home by the patient appears to be an excellent way of overcoming this white coat effect. In 1940, Ayman et al. emphasised the fact that *"the influence of the doctor or the nurse on the patient is significant and it has often been observed in practice that an abrupt or nervous physician will record higher levels than a calm one"*. These authors recommended overcoming the bias by educating the patient to take his own blood pressure at home (or to have it measured by a member of his family) [14].

9. Riva-Rocci S. Un nuovo sfigmomanometro. *Gazzetta Medica di Torino* 1896; 50: 981-996; 51: 1000-1017. — Riva-Rocci S. De la mensuration de la pression artérielle en clinique (On clinical measurement of blood pressure). *Press méd* 1899; 93: 307-308.

10. Potain. *La pression artérielle de l'homme à l'état normal et pathologique* (Blood pressure in health and disease). 1902. Masson, Paris. This work was the first major monograph on blood pressure in clinical medicine.

11. Janeway T.C. *The clinical study of blood pressure.* 1904. D. Appleton & Co., New York and London.

12. Conversely, the lowering of blood pressure which occurred following bed rest during the first days of hospitalisation was recognised. Pancrazio. On the clinical measurement of blood pressure. *Rivista crit di clinica med.* 1908: 2.

13. Deadborn. Practical notes on hypertension. *Medical Record*; September 16, 1916.

14. Ayman D., Goldshine A. Blood pressure determinations by patients with essential hypertension. *Am J Med Sci* 1940; 200: 465-474. The first case of self-measurement appears to be that reported by Brown in 1930; Brown G.E. Daily and monthly rhythm in the blood pressure of a man with hypertension. *Ann Int Med* 1930; 3: 1177.

Gazzetta Medica di Torino

1896: Riva-Rocci's recommendation for measuring blood pressure

In his article published on December 17, 1896 in the *Gazzetta Medica di Torino*, Riva-Rocci made the following recommendation:
"When the patient has been placed in what we believe to be the best position possible (in usual cases, the patient is sitting on the bed), complete rest and absolute calm are indispensable because even the slightest emotion can cause an appreciable disturbance in the level of blood pressure".

Already the problem of hypertension was being extended to a concern with prognosis and treatment. Although Ayman et al. advocated self-measurement, they stated: *"It should be pointed out that our results are not intended to suggest that the one million or more hypertensive patients in the United States should all be buying sphygmomanometers. In practice, self-measurement should, for the time being, be restricted to special cases or to studies on antihypertensive treatment"*. Half a century later, these restrictions are perhaps in the process of disappearing under the commercial pressure of manufacturers of self-measurement devices.

Following on from the earlier recommendations of Basch, Riva-Rocci, Janeway and Gallavardin, the World Health Organisation set forth a series of recommendations for measuring blood pressure. But applying these recommendations in daily clinical practice is still problematical today. The delicate question of the use of the newer ambulatory methods has made the problem even more complex.

THE ERA OF MARGINAL FACTORS:
ALTITUDE, DIGESTION AND MENSTRUATION

At the end of the 19th century, the early use of the manometer revealed the numerous factors that could influence blood pressure and which were the object of intense and very detailed investigation. Thus the ability to measure blood pressure opened up a whole new area of investigation in which certain investigators found themselves lost along paths leading either nowhere or at best to very marginal factors such as altitude, digestion or menstruation [15]. This profusion of marginal studies reflects the absence of epidemiological and clinical data in an era when measurements were made simply out of curosity. The relationship between the instrument and the significance of what it actually measured had not been fully realised and was overshadowed by a fascination with the characteristics of the apparatus itself. It would be true to say that many contributions by Basch and Potain were sometimes restricted to this aspect [16].

In 1887, Basch (cited by Potain) reported that after 10 minutes of rapid mountain climbing his radial pressure rose from 125 to 185 mmHg. To study the influence of atmospheric pressure on blood pressure, Potain performed a series of measurements during excursions in a hot air balloon at an altitude of 315 meters. He climbed the Eiffel Tower and also climbed to an altitude of 1500 metres on Mount Revard. These observations were made in the company of his family, his friends, students or colleagues. To confirm his data, Potain, shut himself, his senior registrar and one of his students in a pneumatic chamber and noted that an increase in external pressure was accompanied by a significant rise in arterial pressure. To refine his observations even

15. Bogdanovics. *Blood pressure in menstruation and delivery.* Orvosi Hetilap; 1909.
Culberston. The study of menopause and related vasomotor disturbances. *Surgery, Gynecology and Obstetrics*; December 1916.
Guillemard and Régnier. Recherches sur la pression artérielle en haute montagne (Research on blood pressure at high altitude). *Société de Biologie;* November 8, 1913.
Loéper. La tension artérielle pendant la digestion (Blood pressure during digestion). *Arch mal coeur;* 1912: 224.

16. Potain certainly deserves credit for being a pioneer of blood pressure measurement in the hospital setting. It would be an exaggeration, however, to say that he fully understood the significance of his own measurements and he certainly did not recognise hypertension as a separate disease entity.

further, he recorded the blood pressure of a young relative travelling from Grenoble to Lyon and observed that the blood pressure rose and fell as the altitude changed! Unfortunately these results were confounded by emotional factors and Potain himself admitted that *"at the start of the journey, the excitement had caused the blood pressure to rise such that the influence of changes in altitude were initially not very apparent"*! After the hot air balloon and the Eiffel Tower, other authors pursued investigations on the influence of altitude using a new technical advance, the aeroplane. Thus, in 1916, Ferry published numerous articles on this subject. But here again, it soon became apparent that blood pressure during flight, take-off or landing were influenced by a decreased oxygen supply, physical exhaustion and emotions [17].

During this pioneering era, the curiosity of investigators knew no bounds. The influence of digestion, menopause and menstruation were all closely examined. Potain studied the blood pressure of 11 subjects after a heavy meal washed down with lots of wine (for once medical students served as guinea-pigs to their advantage!). Potain reported that *"seven of the subjects had an increase in their blood pressure. They were all young male medical students with hearty appetites. Two middle-aged subjects with moderate appetites had a fairly marked lowering of the blood pressure and two, who had eaten very little, had no change at all"*. Less anedoctal was Potain's observations in a subject on an exclusive milk diet whose blood pressure dropped by 20 mmHg after four or five days. Whereas investigations into the influence of digestion on blood pressure resulted in little useful clinical information, the effects of diet were to lead to important therapeutic and pathophysiological advances. These advances were in fact attributable to researchers working on the pathophysiology of hypertension rather than its measurement. Other investigations on the influence of temperature later proved to be of relevance to pyrotherapy, while detailed measurement of blood pressure variations at different times during the menstrual cycle are, today, without any clinical significance.

THE INFLUENCE OF DAY AND NIGHT

The influence of day and night on various disease states has aroused the interest of researchers since the days of Hippocrates and blood pressure was no exception to this rule. The nocturnal drop in blood pressure was noted very early on by several investigators [18]. Gallavardin [19] noted that *"Like all physiological functions (brain activity, muscle tone, temperature, heart rate, etc.) blood pressure undergoes circadian variations"*. As time passed, the increasing sophistication of measuring instruments enabled more accurate studies of circadian variations in blood pressure both in hypertensive and normal subjects and new publications followed each technological innovation. Continuous recordings confirmed and clarified the results of earlier investigators. Beyond simply describing the facts,

17. Ferry. Le syndrome "mal des aviateurs": étude expérimentale de la tension artérielle en vol (The pilot's syndrome; experimental study of blood pressure during flight). *Presse Méd*; February 10, 1916.

18. Mac William J.A. Blood pressure and heart action in sleep and dreams. *Brit Med J;* 1923; 2: 1196.
Brooks H., Carroll K.H. A clinical study of the effects of sleep and rest on blood pressure. *Arch Intern Med* 1912; 10: 97.
Brush C.E. , Fairweather R. Observations on the changes in blood pressure during normal sleep. *Am J Physiol* 1901; 5: 199.
Hill L. Arterial pressure in man while sleeping, resting, working, bathing. *Physiol* 1898; 72: 26-29.

19. Gallavardin L. *La Tension artérielle en clinique* (Blood pressure in clinical practice). 1920. Masson, Paris.

investigators began to wonder about the prognostic significance of inversions of the circadian cycle observed in certain individuals. Changes, or an inversion of the circadian cycle raised difficult diagnostic and prognostic questions in patients with severe hypertension, renal insufficiency, Cushing's syndrome, or in extreme cases of sleep apnoea. Recent cross-sectional studies have shown that the absence of a nocturnal drop in blood pressure and, in extreme cases, the inversion of the circadian cycle are associated with an elevation of the left ventricular mass index (on echocardiography) and a higher incidence of cerebral lesions (CAT-scan or MRI). Modern longitudinal studies appear to confirm that an inversion of the circadian cycle is a poor prognostic factor in terms of both morbidity and mortality. There is some evidence that an inversion of the circadian cycle in cases of pregnancy-associated hypertension may be of predictive value and could herald the onset of eclampsia. A new typology of patients has even been suggested. It is this day-night difference which has led to the differenciation of so-called dippers and non-dippers [20].

Studies on exercise and age-related changes in blood pressure were also undertaken very early and are important because of their diagnostic, nosological and therapeutic implications [21]. Many articles were written about the increase in blood pressure with age which raised the difficult problem of what is normal and what is abnormal. An additional difficulty was that this age-related increase in hypertension made it difficult to evaluate new treatments. The haemodynamic consequences of *"senile ridigity of the arteries"*, already alluded to by Marey in the 19th century, continues to be the subject of many studies today.

MEASURING TO PREDICT

In the early 1960s, M. Sokolow and his co-workers began using portable recorders and attributed prognostic significance to their findings. They showed that among patients with comparable casual blood pressure recordings, those who had higher ambulatory values or those who had prolonged elevation were more likely to have organic lesions such as left ventricular hypertrophy on ECG or abnormalities on examination of the fundus. Such patients were also more likely to have a history of cardiovascular accidents [22].

These authors thus showed that ambulatory recording improved the prognostic value of blood pressure, which was no longer simply a snapshot but now reflected changes over time. Ayman had clearly recognised this a quarter of a century before when he wrote: *"Blood pressure determinations by patients at home would be useful to inform patients about the nature of their disease to help the physicians to observe the natural course of the disease and to permit clear-cut evaluation of treatment"* [23].

20. O'Brien E., Sheridan J., O'Malley K. Dippers and non dippers. *Lancet* 1988; 13: 397.

21. Middleton. The influence of athletic training on blood pressure. *Am. J. Med. Sci.*; September 1915. Pachon. Education physique et critères fonctionnels: la variation de la pression artérielle, critères d'entraînement (Physical education and functional criteria; variations in blood pressure as a criterion for training). *Société de biologie*, May 21 and 23, 1910.
Wildt. Blood pressure in elderly subjects. *Zentralbl. F. Herz u. Gefässkr*, February 1912.

22. Kain H.K., Hinman A.T., Sokolow M. Arterial blood pressure measurements with a portable recorder in hypertensive patients. I. Variability and correlation with casual pressure. *Circulation* 1964; 30: 882-892.

23. Ayman D., Goldshine A. Blood pressure determinations by patients with essential hypertension. *Am J Med Sci* 1940; 200: 465-474.

Marking blood pressure with a red pencil:
The sphygmomanometer enters the operating theatre.

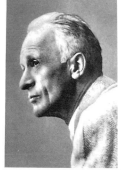

At the turn of the century, Harvey Cushing (1869-1939) (top)) was already insisting that all his surgical patients have their heart rate and respiratory rate recorded on a chart during operation. In 1901 he travelled to Europe where he met Riva-Rocci and Mosso who aroused his interest in the measurement of blood pressure. On his return, he recommended the measurement of blood pressure during operation. In 1904 Theodore Janeway credited Cushing with this innovation:

"Systematic measurement of the blood pressure during operation is being widely adopted by surgeons, and bids fair to become general. It may easily be carried out by the anesthesist. To be of a value, a determination should be made every five minutes, and, with the pulse rate, recorded on a chart which can be seen by the operator. This procedure was originally recommended by Cushing. The chart described heretofore is well adapted for the purpose, and is more easily read if the systolic pressure be marked with a red pencil, the pulse in blue or black" (below).

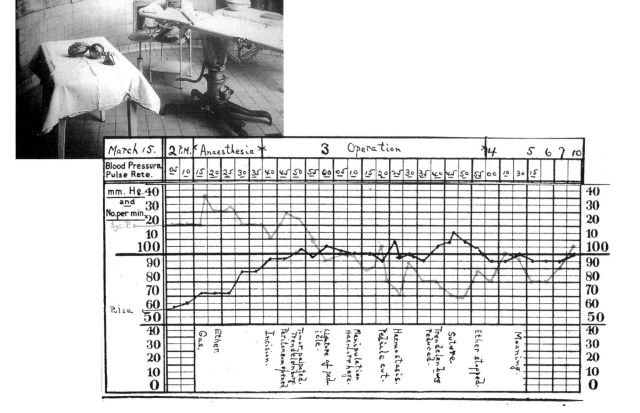

Chart reproduced from Janeway's book: *The clinical study of blood pressure, a guide to use the sphygmomanometer in medical, surgical, and obstetrical practice with a summary of the experimental and clinical facts relating to the blood pressure in health and disease.* 1904. D. Appleton and Company, New York and London.

Blood pressure determinations were soon to enter the realm of diagnosis [24]. Publications on the measurement of hypertension had a bright future and, in recognition of its potential, a journal devoted to hypertension was started. With the study of short-term variations, made possible by the availability of new tools, a whole new field of investigations is opening up for clinicians. Will the results of these studies lead to new diagnostic and therapeutic applications ? Will traditional blood pressure recordings performed in the doctor's office soon be completely obsolete ? Only the future will tell.

24. Today, the study of short-term variations using spectral analysis or also assessment of the baroreflex is a useful diagnostic tool for demonstrating autonomic dysfunction or an alteration in the regulation of the baroreflex arc. This is of practical importance in the presence of manifestations such as malaise, syncope or as a routine procedure in patients prone to sympathetic or parasympathetic disturbances, such as diabetics. The value of this analysis is now clearly established except in hypertensive patients with cardiac failure.

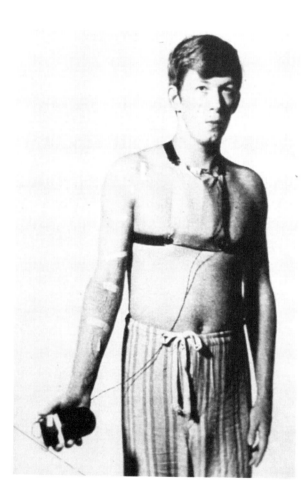

The Oxford intra-arterial system for 24-hour blood pressure measurement. Reproduced from: Pickering G. High blood pressure, 2nd ed. 1968. J & A Churchill, London.

Direct intra-arterial recording

The idea of recording variations in blood pressure is an old one. In the middle of the 19th century, Ludwig produced the first continuous recordings in dogs using his sphygmograph. The blood pressure was recorded by means of a stylet on smoke-blackened paper. In the 1960s, the first truly portable recorders usable in man made their appearance thanks in particular to the contributions of the Oxford group. In 1966, Bevan and his co-workers developed a new system for direct intra-arterial measurements. This invasive method provided a very detailed and complete study of blood pressure variations.

RECOGNISING HYPERTENSION

The essential contribution of life insurance companies to the discovery of risk

"If it is true that certain statisticians know little about medicine, it is unfortunately even more true that most physicians know little or nothing about statistics. This is one of the great lessons to be learnt from the insurance companies".

M. Loéper
2nd International Congress of Life Insurance Physicians
Paris. May 18-21, 1939.

Physicians working for life insurance companies were the first to suspect, and then to demonstrate that hypertension was a major cardiovascular risk factor. This essential contribution was not due to chance. It was the result of almost a century of work calculating the life expectancy of individuals. It is noteworthy that the emergence of the concept of hypertension as a risk factor had little, if anything, to do with experimental and pathophysiological preoccupations. Thus, it was neither the inventors of the instruments nor the clinicians who reaped the first practical rewards of the early work on hypertension, but physicians working for life insurance companies. Even before the first clinically usable apparatus became available, life-insurance physicians were already using the stethoscope and the sphygmograph to try to calculate, as accurately as they could, the life expectancy of people taking out life-insurance policies. In addition to this innovative use of new investigational tools, they proved to be the most competent and active in setting up large-scale epidemiological studies, in North America in particular.

Financial transactions with the family of the deceased are nothing new. Already in the 15th century, certain marriage contracts made provision for compensation of families in the case of the loss of a spouse. Similarly, maritime insurance companies in Antwerp were offering their passengers life insurance as far back as the 16th century. In the 16th and 17th centuries, certain insurance policies appeared here and there, prefiguring the future life insurance policies. But they were looked upon as a wager on death and were considered immoral and therefore forbidden because it was felt that they could encourage the beneficiary of the policy to wish for the death of the insured [1].

1. As far back as the 16th century, maritime insurance companies in Antwerp offered life insurance policies to their passengers. In the 17th century, the Napolitan banker Lorenzo Totti proposed a system of life annuity in which the capital was distributed to the survivors, thus inaugurating the tontine system, which was not forbidden.

Later, and for many years, the first life insurance policies had to face the prejudice of potential policy purchasers who feared that by signing a contract, they were "signing their own death warrant" [2].

In was in England during the second half of the 18th century that life insurance really made its appearance to "*prevent misery, preserve the well-being of families and prepare for a happy and peaceful old-age*" in the words of a banker of the time [3]. In the years that followed, other companies sprung up all over Europe, fostered by the expansion of capitalism. By the decade 1820-1830, life insurance existed as we know it today, but it was not until the latter part of the century that it really underwent rapid development. In 1874, there were something like 200 insurance companies with over a million policy holders [4].

CALCULATING THE STATISTICS OF FATE

To insure an individual's life meant calculating how much time he had left to live. Calculating life expectancy was difficult. The question had been considered as far back as Hippocrates, when an attempt was made to establish prognoses in various diseases, but the concept of a numerical estimation of life expectancy in healthy subjects emerged only in the 17th century. Insurance policy premiums indexed on age made their appearance in England back in 1720. With the help of a physician, Dr Price, a London insurance company used actuarial calculations to determine its premiums in 1762. This calculation required the use of longevity tables or rather "mortality tables" which the British, no doubt of more naturally optimistic disposition, called life tables [5]. For many years, French life insurance companies used the tables of Deparcieux and Duvillard which were established in the 18th century and were the only ones available apart from that of Buffon. Thus, a financial report of the Royal Insurance Company states: "*According to Buffon and Deparcieux, the total combined number of deaths amongst policy holders will be 1,721 and they will cost the company £3,000 each*" [3].

Initially, the calculations were basic and very approximate because the tables were essentially a registry in which the duration of life for any given group was simply listed. These tables provided no more than an indication of the mortality in the general population. As time went by, the young science of statistics made a truly probabilistic approach possible, and mortality tables became "*probability tables on human life*" [6]. Laplace thus calculated "*the mean duration of life*" which he presented as "*life expectancy in the mathematical sense of the term*". He went one step further by emphasising the mathematical criteria which needed to be met to guarantee reliable interpretation. In his own words: "*One can conceive that the accuracy of these results*

2. First international congress of life insurance physicians. Opening session. Brussels 1899.

3. Commemoration of the centenary of "La Nationale" (non commercial edition). Albert Morangé Publishers, 1930. In France, on February 10, 1787, the financier Beaufleury (who headed a fire insurance company), acting on behalf of "*a company of well-known citizens whose goal was more to make itself useful than to earn large profits*" proposed to create "*an establishment that no-one had hitherto thought of*". He submitted the "*principles and calculations for the setting up of a human life insurance company*" to the baron de Breteuil who was then minister to the King. The privilege was granted in 1787. Some consideration was given to limiting this privilege to a period of 15 years. It was argued, however, that while each person's life must come to an end, life itself is endless.

4. Davis A.B., *Medicine and its technology: an introduction to the history of medical instrumentation.* 1981, Greenwood Press.

5. Although a mortality table attributed to Ulpien in 1364 is sometimes cited, it appears that the first real table of this type was that of John Graunt, a London merchant and Major in the police force of his city. It was published in 1661. Other tables followed, namely the "extinction table" of Jacob van Daël (1670) and the mortality table by the Dutchman Jean De Witt (1671). A large number of such tables appeared in the 18th century and were used particularly for the calculation of life annuities.

6. Buffon used the term "table of probability" but he did not really apply any sophisticated mathematical calculation to it. The concept of probability was pioneered in the 17th century by Pascal, Roberval and Fernet. At the turn of the 19th century, Laplace made a major

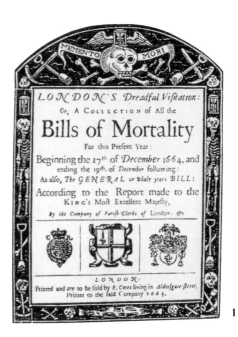

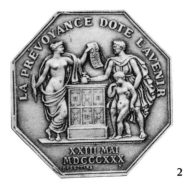

2

The inscription on the French life insurance company medallion reads "Providence endows the future". 1830.

1

A 19th century poster caricaturing insurance companies. The poster reads "Insurance against insurance".

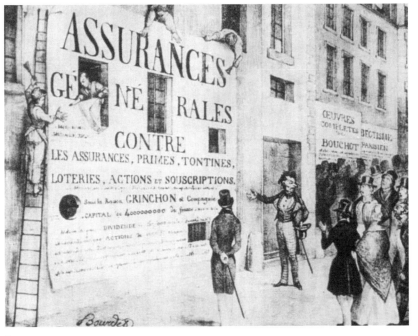

3

Life insurance physicians: the pioneers of research on "obscure diseases"

Physicians working for life insurance companies made an essential contribution to the recognition of hypertension as a risk factor. From 1850 to 1900, that is before blood pressure was measured in man — a noteworthy fact — this group of physicians displayed remarkable foresight in studying "obscure diseases" by the clinical and investigational methods available to them at the time. As early as 1907 they were the first to foresee the prognostic potential of measuring blood pressure in asymptomatic individuals, and by 1920, they had come up with statistics on large groups of hypertensive patients. This remarkable work was not due to chance but was the result of long experience. The early mortality tables dating back to the 17th century (*figure 1*) were completely revised by insurance companies after medical selection of their potential clients. Because of their popularity and commercial success (*figures 2 and 3*), insurance companies were able to devote the necessary resources to show that hypertension played an important role in cardiovascular morbidity and mortality.

requires a very large number of births; the analysis of probabilities shows that the results come closer and closer to the truth, and finally coincide with reality when the number of births considered reaches infinity" [7].

The study of longevity was entering an era of dynamic analysis. In 1835, Quetelet evaluated *"the influence of the development of civilisation and standard of living"* which had decreased the annual probability of dying from 1/30 to 1/40. The study of probabilities and the progress of statistics put a mathematical slant on the duration of human life which was *"of the utmost importance for physicians and administrators"*, Laplace rightly emphasised. Insurance companies quickly realised the limits of statistics based on church registries or figures from city or state registry offices and so they put together their own mortality tables. This approach was an innovative form of medical statistics because it was based on a selected sample. It was in the anglo-saxon countries, pioneers in the field of insurance, that the new statistical approach emerged and developed, while in France, jealous custodian of its clinical *"savoir-faire"* there was a tendency to ignore the influence of numerical analysis in medicine, despite the brilliant contribution of Louis [8]. The first table based on the experience of an insurance company, rather than on general mortality, was published in 1778 by Charles Brand on the basis of 3,826 deaths.

EVALUATING INDIVIDUAL RISK

In the early days of life insurance, while mortality tables were the only reference point for calculating life expectancy, insurance agents quickly recognised that certain categories of individuals, those in the armed forces in particular, did not conform to the statistics of the general population because of their occupational risk. These categories were therefore not eligible for life insurance. Similarly, death resulting from a duel or from suicide was considered to be grounds for non-payment of compensation. These cases of exclusion represented an early attempt to recognise individual risk, though they were based on social rather than medical criteria. But disease was of course the major factor influencing longevity and the concept of "natural", as opposed to "disease-related" death came into being [9].

Starting in the middle of the 19th century, insurance agents learned to take account of the medical environment of the contracting parties. Those who lived in insalubrious regions of the colonies were required to pay higher premiums because of what was called a "tropical risk" [10]. Likewise, cholera, which was prevalent at that time, was also given special mention. Life insurance provided the impetus for a statistical analysis of life expectancy in "healthy" individuals.

mathematical contribution and showed how probabilities could be applied to the human sciences, for example for calculating life expectancy.

7. Laplace, 10th lesson on probabilities, 1795, in *Oeuvres* (Works), volume XIV, p.168. As early as 1783, Laplace alluded to the importance of random sampling for obtaining representative samples.

8. Piquemal J., Succès et décadence de la méthode numérique en France à l'époque de Pierre-Alexandre Louis (The rise and fall of the numerate method in France at the time of Pierre-Alexandre Louis) in *Essais et leçons d'histoire de la médecine et de la biologie* (Essays and lessons in medicine and biology), 1993, Presses Universitaires de France, Paris.

9. Several years after Laplace, Cournot raised the issue of differentiating statistically between "natural" and "disease-related" death: *"If a living being could escape all accidental causes of destruction resulting from either sudden and violent death or from disease leading to death after a more or less prolonged period, one would observe the natural duration of life"*. Cournot, 1843. *Exposition de la théorie des chances et des probabilités* (On the theory of chance and probability). Chapter XIII, section 171, pp. 310-312.

10. Yellow fever in particular.

E LONDON CHARIVARI. 137

PIUIAHL
ASSURANCE COI
CAPITAL : 150

parle.
:kless
s the
wick,
iently
n the
ime a
tually
:h till

BBLE-
.E im-
t with
play,
is one
dded.
y the
posed
:d for
He,
l this
he. I
s I do
oblest
)dious
nities.
bling-
iendly
what
refer-
of his

', sug-
grasp
smoky
very
gaged
s hat.
obody
)ffered
Pas si
Lady

Per-
:d note
:k her
lid not

Doctor. "Now, what did your Father and Mother die of?"
Applicant. "Well, Sir, I can't say as I do 'xactly remember; but 'twarn't nothing serious!"

cultural Society. These ladies looked wickedly nice in grass lawn and lace, which Mrs. PLANTAGENET-NIBBS—who is always inclined to be nasty—said would give their mothers no trouble

Early attempts to identify vascular risk

Early attempts to evaluate risk in medicine were the work of the life insurance companies. Founded in Europe in the 18th century, life insurance companies really prospered in the United States. In 1874 some 200 North American companies had issued over a million life insurance policies. This provided them with access to clinical and statistical material far beyond the reach of the medical establishment.

As shown in this cartoon which appeared in the British press, the "Bourgeoisie" was well aware of the inquisitive attitude of the insurance company doctor who performed a thorough examination and took a full history.

(Wood engraving by L.G. Raven Hill, 1896)

It was Fischer, medical director of the Northwestern Mutual Life Insurance Company, who first included the measurement of blood pressure in the examination of life insurance applicants around 1905. At the time, doctors knew nothing of the prognostic value of blood pressure and its measurement had not yet been adopted into everyday medical practice. Even Theodore Janeway, a pioneer in the field of hypertension, wrote in 1913: *"The relation of the height of the blood pressure to prognosis is doubtful. [...] The exact height of the blood pressure does not seem to have much bearing on the expectancy of life. The average duration of life in this group of patients, after the onset of symptoms associated with high blood pressure, has been four years for the men and five for the women. One-half of the whole number of deceased died during the first five years. One-quarter of the number lived between five and ten years, and the remaining quarter over ten years from the appearance of the first symptom. The existence of this considerable number of patients living for a long period of time suggests the need of great caution in making a prognosis as to expectancy of life".* The tide began to turn with the publication of the "Report of the Committee on Blood Pressure", at the instigation of the life insurance companies, in 1917.

Mortality and apoplexy: early indications in the 17th century

In London in the 17th century, the first attempts at descriptive epidemiology were represented by the Bills of Mortality. Cases of apoplexy were mentioned, suggesting complications of hypertension, though with great uncertainty. The major killer in the large cities however, was infection. But by the mid-19th century the death registries maintained by the insurance companies (on selected individuals not representative of the general population) began to reveal the growing importance of apoplexy — even though the sphygmomanometer had not yet been invented.

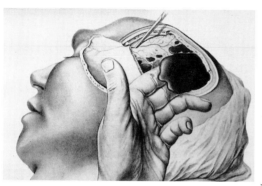

Natural and *Political*

OBSERVATIONS

Mentioned in a following INDEX,

and made upon the

Bills of Mortality.

By *JOHN GRAUNT*,

Citizen of

LONDON.

With reference to the *Government*, *Religion*, *Trade*, *Growth*, *Ayre*, *Diseases*, and the several Changes of the said CITY.

—— *Non, me ut miretur Turba, laboro,*
Contentus paucis Lectoribus ——

LONDON,
Printed by *Tho: Roycroft*, for *John Martin*, *James Allestry*, and *Tho: Dicas*, at the Sign of the *Bell* in St. *Paul's* Church-yard, MDCLXII.

The *Diseases*, and *Casualties* this year being 1632.

Abortive, and Stilborn — 445	Jaundies — 43
Affrighted — 1	Jawfaln — 8
Aged — 628	Impostume — 74
Ague — 43	Kil'd by several accidents — 46
Apoplex, and Meagrom — 17	King's Evil — 38
Bit with a mad dog — 1	Lethargie — 2
Bleeding — 3	Livergrown — 87
Bloody flux, scowring, and flux 348	Lunatique — 5
Brused, Issues, sores, and ulcers, 28	Made away themselves — 15
Burnt, and Scalded — 5	Measles — 80
Burst, and Rupture — 9	Murthered — 7
Cancer, and Wolf — 10	Over-laid, and starved at nurse — 7
Canker — 1	Palsie — 25
Childbed — 171	Piles — 1
Chrisomes, and Infants — 2268	Plague — 8
Cold, and Cough — 55	Planet — 13
Colick, Stone, and Strangury — 56	Pleurisie, and Spleen — 36
Consumption — 1797	Purples, and spotted Feaver — 38
Convulsion — 241	Quinsie — 7
Cut of the Stone — 5	Rising of the Lights — 98
Dead in the street, and starved — 6	Sciatica — 1
Dropsie, and Swelling — 267	Scurvey, and Itch — 9
Drowned — 34	Suddenly — 62
Executed, and prest to death — 18	Surfet — 86
Falling Sicknes — 7	Swine Pox — 6
Fever — 1108	Teeth — 470
Fistula — 13	Thrush, and Sore mouth — 40
Flocks, and small Pox — 531	Tympany — 13
French Pox — 12	Tissick — 34
Gangrene — 5	Vomiting — 1
Gout — 4	Worms — 27
Grief — 11	

Christened	Males — 4994	Buried	Males — 4932		Whereof,
	Females - 4590		Females — 4603		of the
	In all — 9584		In all — 9535		Plague 8

Increased in the Burials in the 122 Parishes, and at the Pesthouse this year   993
Decreased of the Plague in the 122 Parishes, and at the Pesthouse this year,   266

Then, at the turn of the 20th century, comparisons began to be made between normal and "defective" individuals which led to the calculation of an "increased risk", a concept which was eventually to usher in a new era of preventive medicine.

Insurance companies began to tailor their contracts to the state of health of their clients. In other words, they began selecting their clients, initially to exclude those who had a physical or hereditary defect judged to be too severe. For "*such a necessary and difficult selection, no one could replace the physician*" [11]. Neither the demographer, nor the economist, nor the hygienist could replace the physician who was the only one qualified to look for and detect pathological factors that could predict an asymptomatic disease. "*The intervention of the physician appears quite natural in a financial operation based on the probable duration of human life from any point in time*", stated a treatise on life insurance published in 1887 [11]. The certified medical expert had thus come into existence [12].

LOOKING FOR "OBSCURE DISEASES": A NEW MISSION FOR THE PHYSICIAN

When physicians working for insurance companies began to look for asymptomatic disorders, then called "obscure diseases", they were making an important step because they were, unknowingly, inventing a new approach to medicine. For the first time, physicians were examining individuals who came to them not because they had symptoms, but for economic reasons. The objective here was not to treat but to question, to observe and to examine with a view to making a "*previsional diagnosis*" to use the expression of Vleminckx, president of the first congress of insurance company physicians held in Brussels in 1899. Here was a novel mission for the physician who, apart from the recruitment of conscripts into the Army, had not hitherto been accustomed to dealing with healthy individuals who came to be examined rather than treated. Thus came into being the first "examining physicians" as the insurance companies called them back in 1832. Their role has become increasingly important ever since. With them, came a new "*science of diagnosis and prognosis*", to use the expression of Vleminckx.

In 1824, for the first time, a medical service was attached to an insurance company, the Clerical Medical and General, and in 1839 the German company La Gotha followed suit. In 1858 , the Equitable Company in England appointed a medical examiner. His major task was to design a questionnaire to be filled in by the examining physician for each applicant. This relentless pursuit of information, continually improved by the experience of previous years and sometimes performed in collaboration with physicians from other companies, gradually built up a valuable epidemiological resource.

11. Anonymous. *Traité complet de l'examen médical dans les assurances de la vie* (Complete treatise of medical examination in life insurance). 1887. L. Warnier , Paris. The author of this anonymous treatise is believed to be Dr Mauriac, judging by the tribute he was paid at the first international congress of life insurance physicians in Brussels in 1899.

12. According to Ingman, the first physicians to work for life insurance companies were in Scotland in 1811. Ingman H.W. *Insurability, prognosis and selection.* 1927. The Spectator Company. Chicago, New York.

The insurance company physician's objective was not to relieve suffering, but to devote all his efforts to a detailed search for personal and family history and to record anthropometric data. Like modern epidemiologists, the insurance company physician was in an ideal position to study certain statistical questions of the upmost importance from a medical standpoint, and particularly to determine the probability that an applicant would stay alive. As we will see later, insurance agents proved to be better than clinicians at determining risk factors.

By the end of the 19th century, all the major insurance companies had adopted the use of very detailed medical questionnaires combined with a medical examination. Highly qualified physicians were hired for this work and they gathered together important statistical data. *"No other administration could be in a position to collect such information on the family and personal history of an individual, his temperament, his profession, his lifestyle, his position of wealth and, of course finally the cause of death"* [11]. In 1832, the questionnaire of *La Nationale* insurance company included specific questions on the presence of *"epilepsy, paralysis or mental alienation, headaches, frequent colds, spitting of blood and asthma with palpitation"* [3]. Twenty years later, most European and North American companies were using very detailed questionnaires that sought to detect virtually every disease affecting man. Because they were so exhaustive in their approach, these documents were far more relevant and valuable than the case reports of hospital clinicians. *"In accuracy, there is no comparison between the statistical documents of insurance companies and similar documents taken from hospital surveys or registries"* [11]. There was general agreeement on the usefulness of statistical data from insurance companies and on the shortcomings of hospital registries.

UNDER SCRUTINY BY THE STETHOSCOPE AND THE SPHYGMOGRAPH

With an historically new mission in medicine, the insurance company physician's role had become to *"discover the major prognostic signs of obscure diseases"* [11]. He was guided in this new role by the anatomico-clinical method championed by Corvisart, Bichat and Laënnec of the Paris School of Medicine. The method sought to establish a link between symptoms and specific organ alterations. But here there were no symptoms. The clinical examination became a routine procedure which aimed to detect silent or so-called "latent" alterations with a view to determining the probable lifespan of an insurance policy applicant. By pursuing this historically new statistical objective — that is to calculate the probable lifespan of groups of medically selected individuals — insurance company doctors created a new medical specialty on the fringe of the traditional medical establishment. In 1889, the medical directors of life insurance companies

The statistics from the life insurance companies speak for themselves

In 1917, Dr Fischer, who pioneered the inclusion of blood pressure measurement in the medical examination of life insurance applicants, presented his report of the diagnostic value of the systolic blood pressure covering the period from August 1 1907 to August 1 1915. This 8-year follow-up data on subjects aged 40 to 60 years led him to state that *"the higher the arterial tension, the greater the mortality"*. His work is summed up by 7 main conclusions:

I.   That a persistently high arterial tension will result in an excessive mortality, and the higher the arterial tension, the greater the mortality.

II. That a persistent systolic blood pressure of about 12 mm above the average for the age would seem to indicate the limit of normal excess variation in man.

III. That an apparently healthy person may have high arterial tension, extending over a considerable period of time without a discoverable impairment to account for same.

IV. That of the medical impairments found, together with high arterial tension, both below and above the age of 40, more than 75 per cent are cardiovascular.

V.   That while the normal average blood pressure increases with age so far as investigated (i.e., age 60 or 65), materially higher arterial tension is not necessarily to be expected at older ages.

VI. That persons with a systolic blood pressure between 90 to 110 mm show a more favorable mortality than persons with a pressure 12 mm above the average pressure for the age.

VII. That in persons whose weight is 20 per cent or more in excess of the average for height and age, blood pressure averages about 4 mm higher than those of normal weight.

The synoptic table below shows that beyond a systolic pressure of 170 mmHg the risk exceeds 200%. These subjects were rejected for life insurance and appear in the REJ'TD column.

Source: Abstracts of the proceedings of the Association of Life Insurance Medical Directors of America (1917).

Summary of the Mortality Experience of the N.W. Mut. Life Ins. Co., with respect to Systolic Blood Pressure.

Period	No. Risks Acc'd	No. Risks Rej'td	Ages (inc)	B.P. Mm.Hg. Range	B.P. Mm.Hg. Av.	Other Impt.	Mortality to Aug 1 1915 (M.A. Table)	%
Aug. 1 1907 to Aug. 1 1910	2630		40-60	140-149	142	—		93 16
	521		40-60	150-160	152⁵	—		127 00
		302	40-60		170	None.		250 41
		288	40-60		171	One or More.		302 16
Aug. 1 1907 to Aug. 1 1915		1274	40-60		160	None.		220 11
		956	40-60		165	One or More.		263 76
Nov. 1911 Aug. 1915		495	16-39		150	None.		142 61
Low B.P. 1907-1910 (inc)	200		40-60	105 & under		—		47 00
	427		40-60	106-110		—		65 00
Low B.P. Nov 1911 to Aug. 1915.	433		16-39	100 & under		—	2 Deaths.	
		60	40-60			—	No Deaths.	

joined forces in the *Association of Life Insurance Medical Directors of America* and in the decade 1870-1880 new specialised journals began to appear. A new form of epidemiology, privately inspired, had come into being. Its quality, efficacy and reliability were guaranteed by a most powerful factor: the financial interests of the bankers.

After taking a careful and detailed history, the physician examined the applicant — and not the patient — taking particular care to look for signs suggestive of the major diseases of the time: syphilis, phtisis, rheumatism, neuropathy and alcoholism. This procedure required *"a detailed knowledge of physiology, anatomy, pathology, clinical examination, biological chemistry and internal medicine"* [2]. Very early on, the physician used a *"diagnostic armamentarium"* which included not only the stethoscope, the basic instrument, but also things like scales, the thermometer, the speculum and also chemical analysis of the urine (detection of pus, albumin, phosphates, urea and uric acid). Also used were examination of the fundus, spirometry and sphygmography (the sphygmograph applied to the wrist provided a graphic representation of the arterial pulse waves). The insurance company physician showed more interest for the use of new diagnostic instruments than the traditional clinician [13]. As early as 1875, the sphygmograph and the spirometer were used in medical examinations by certain insurance companies.

13. Jeannel M. *Arsenal du diagnostic médical* (The armamentarium for medical diagnosis). Doctoral thesis. 1873. Paris.

THE MOST COMMON FORMS OF HEART DISEASE ARE THOSE OF WHICH THE PATIENT IS UNAWARE

In the second half of the 19th century, although the concept of hypertension did not yet exist, the notion of vascular risk was emerging. Insurance company physicians particularly feared cerebral apoplexy (well-identified by the anatomico-clinical method), cardiac failure, rhythm disturbances and above all arteriosclerosis [14]. Vascular sclerosis was a real obsession for the cardiologists of the 19th century. Indeed, not only was it well identified by the scalpel of the morbid anatomists, but it also fell within the broader scope of preoccupation with multiple forms of degeneration described during this century. These included degeneration of the vessels but also of society and of the race (alcoholism and syphilis were considered to be the common denominator of all three).

14. Initially, the term "apoplexy" described all diseases which caused "a sudden loss of consciousness and movements followed by a certain degree of paralysis". Later, a distinction was made between cerebral, pulmonary, or meningeal apoplexy.

The heart and blood vessels were thus the object of very careful examination because insurance company physicians understood that cardiovascular disease was a major cause of death in individuals who were not affected by tuberculosis or syphilis. Even before the conquest of bacterial infections by the antibiotic revolution, the risk of death from cardiovascular disease was well understood. *"I consider the good conditions of the heart and blood vessels to be the best guarantee*

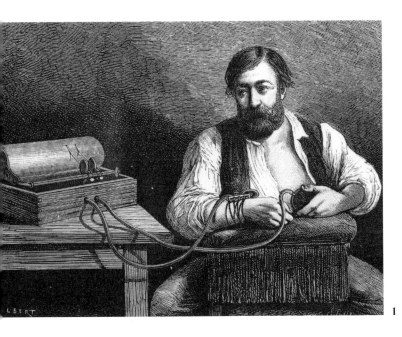

1

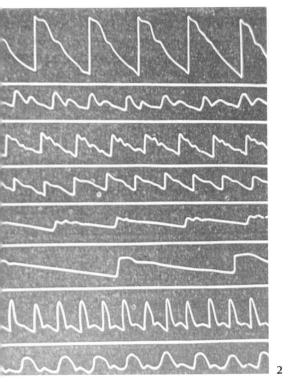

2

The early use of instruments in cardiovascular medicine

The sphygmograph may be considered as the first instrument used in cardiology (*figure 1*). Marey himself recognised that while this device was unable to measure blood pressure, it was useful for the study of rhythm disturbances, valve disease or arteriosclerosis. The pulse waves recorded directly by the sphygmograph provided a new approach to symptomatology as a function of the appearance of what was called the "sphygmogram" (*figure 2*). "1. Senile pulse with cardiac enlargement. - 2. The pulse in typhoid fever. - 3. Lead colic. - 4. Pericarditis. - 5. Convalescence. - 6. Rare senile pulse. - 7. Hectic fever. - 8. Dissecting aneurysm of the aorta."
It is important to note that in the second half of the 18th century, life insurance physicians were the first to use the sphygmometer with the aim of detecting asymptomatic cardiac and vascular disease. This long experience probably explains why they were also the first to generalise the use of the sphygmomanometer in asymptomatic populations.

From E.J. Marey. *La circulation du sang à l'état physiologique et dans les maladies* (Blood circulation in health and disease). 1881, Paris.

of a long life and their degeneration as one of the main causes of premature death" explained Dr Moritz in his presentation on the examination of the heart at the first congress of insurance company physicians [15]. Apoplexy and post-infectious valve lesions were the conditions most commonly encountered, whereas lesions due to *"latent coronary sclerosis are not common enough to cause significant losses to insurance companies"*. However, at the end of the 19th century, there was still considerable confusion between rheumatic heart disease (i.e. post-infectious) and degenerative disease. It was not until the widespread use of radiology, electrocardiography and the sphygmomanometer in the decade 1910-1920 that the situation was clarified.

The insurance company physician, in his examination of the circulatory system, was on the lookout for a history of rheumatic fever. He was well aware of the severity of the sequelae (valvular heart disease) and if he detected them, his instructions were to refuse the insurance policy. He knew full well that heart disease could *"progress in an absolutely latent fashion"* or present as *"atypical, minor or incomplete forms which can conceal the disease [...]. The most common forms of heart disease are those of which the patient himself is unaware and which often surprise the physician by the discovery of organic lesions which were totally unsuspected"* [11]. Cardiac auscultation, which was able to pick up rhythm disturbances and the murmurs of valve disease, could detect such latent conditions. This examination was very accurate and the questionnaire of the Imperial Life Office Company (around 1875) stated: *"Have you examined the patient by percussion and auscultation beneath his clothes?"*. At about the same time, the questionnaire of the La Gotha Insurance Company included the following points: *"What are the results of examination of the heart and blood circulation?*

(a) position and volume of the heart
(b) rhythm, force and volume of heart beat
(c) the state of heart sounds
(d) frequency and uniformity of arterial beats
(e) bruits in the great arteries and veins of the neck
(f) distension and pulsation of the veins".

In the years 1870 to 1890, the examiner did not have at his disposal any instruments for the clinical measurement of blood pressure (they had not yet been invented). However he did know how to study the loss of arterial compliance which was so often noted on autopsy. To study "generalised arteriosclerosis" the sphygmograph was available to complement a very detailed palpation of the arteries. In the case of arteriosclerosis, the tracing showed a "plateau"

15. Dr Moritz. *De l'examen du coeur en matière d'assurance vie* (On examination of the heart in life insurance). First congress of insurance physicians, Brussels. 1899.

reflecting "the anticipated arterial senility" and "the loss of arterial elasticity" [16]. The significance given to arteriosclerosis came from the information obtained from morbid anatomy which, since the dissections of Morgagni in the previous century, had underlined the pathological importance of hardened arteries.

The anatomico-clinical method had also uncovered cardiac enlargement which the physicians tried to detect by locating the apex beat, coupled with the evaluation of the shape and extent of the area of cardiac dullness. Shortly after x-rays became available, they were also used for this purpose [17].

Detecting cardiac enlargement appears to have paid dividends, as witnessed by the following report in 1887. *"The types of heart disease encountered most frequently amongst the applicants are those which interefere little with their cardiopulmonary function and do not yet seriously endanger general health. The patients themselves are unaware of these conditions which often surprise the physician by the discovery of an unsuspected organic lesion. In such circumstances, the finding of a physical sign must lead to rejecting an applicant who at first sight appeared to fulfill the necessary conditions for acceptance"* [11]. It was precisely these unsuspected signs that were targeted by the medical examinations of the insurance companies.

Applicants for life insurance were also routinely screened for albuminuria. If the test was positive, the applicant was rejected. It was known that this abnormality of the urinary sediment could be indicative of Bright's disease, a renal disorder affecting the heart by a poorly understood mechanism and which was to be the object of intense study in investigations on hypertension in the 20th century. In 1899, that is before the concept of hypertension was well established, the insurance company physicians already knew that *"it is important to carefully examine the arteries and particularly the aorta and the heart in patients with albuminuria"*. This practical recommendation was even justified by an attempt at physiological explanation: *"It is perfectly obvious that this albuminuria must be dependent upon blood pressure, although this is difficult to demonstrate. I have tried in the following manner: taking a few individuals without albuminuria, I have placed on their abdomens a tightly-applied cushion on awakening and asked them to keep it in place all day. When I examined their urine in the evening, I found small amounts of albumin"*, explained Dr Moritz during a discussion on the acceptability of subjects with albuminuria [15]. A most relevant remark in the light of what we now know of the relationship between albuminuria and blood pressure.

16. The sphygmograph was invented by Etienne Jules Marey who perfected the work of the German physiologists. This apparatus was the ancestor of instrumentation in cardiology. As far back as 1875, one can find recommendations for its use in examining life insurance applicants.

17. For the evolution of ideas on left ventricular hypertrophy, see chapter 7 — Yesterday's sufferers, today's patients.

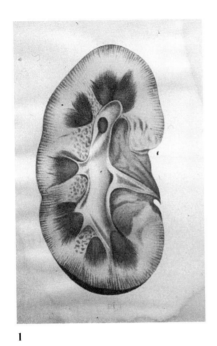

2

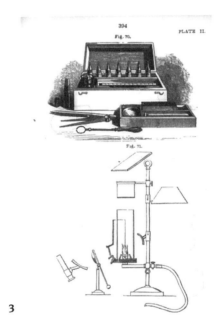

1

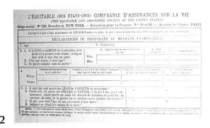

3

Albuminuria, predicting risk before the concept of arterial pressure

In an anatomico-clinical study which has become famous, Richard Bright noted, in 1836, that certain kidney diseases with albuminuria were accompanied by cardiac enlargement. In his original publication, he used the term "pressure" but in a very different sense to the current concept of hypertension. The novel observation of Bright should not be interpreted too broadly by historians of medicine. With remarkable foresight, insurance company physicians used very specific questionnaires (*figure 2*) in the second half of the 19th century and they interpreted albuminuria as a risk factor to be detected by routine assays (*figure 3*).

HYPERTENSION AS AN EXAMPLE
OF THE SUCCESS OF GROUP STUDIES

The invention of instruments for measuring blood pressure originated from advances in experimental medicine rather than from an extension of the anatomico-clinical method. Insurance company physicians quickly recognised the relevance of this invention to their own sphere of interest. It was they who began measuring blood pressure routinely and in doing so, accumulated valuable data. In contrast, hospital records were not well adapted to this type of observation, as was already remarked by insurance companies at the end of the 19th century. This fact also struck Theodore Janeway who, together with his father, was one of the pioneers of the follow-up of hypertensive patients. He noted *"for a satisfactory study of prognosis, only such private material can be used. A study of symptoms from hospital records is so defective as to be of little value. In the first place, ward patients are largely unintelligent and unobservant, and early symptoms are apt to pass unnoticed. In the second place, hospital historians are inexperienced and vary greatly in their ability and the care with which they interrogate the patients. Finally, it would be practically impossible in our hospitals to obtain more than one fraction of the subsequent information which I have been able to collect about these patients"* [18].

In the 1830s, once again well before the introduction of the concept of hypertension, insurance company physicians were already emphasising the importance of death due to "apoplexy", particularly in obese patients. Their long-standing interest in arteriosclerosis predestined them to be the ones to identify vascular risk factors. Their privileged position for the long-term follow-up of patients and their motivation for identifying the medical factors which threatened their clients' future prepared them intellectually for the use of the sphygmomanometer even before it was invented! [19].

According to Scholtz [20], the first study on arterial pressure published in an American journal was that of Howell and Brush in The Boston Medical and Surgical Journal of June 1901. In 1903 in the United States, Theodore Janeway, a physician in private practice, began to measure routinely the blood pressure of his patients. This was a pioneering step. Shortly thereafter, from about 1906 on, Fischer, medical director of the North Western Mutual Life Insurance Company began to take an interest in measuring blood pressure as part of the medical examination of applicants for life insurance. It is precisely to that period 1906-1910 that one can trace the beginnings of the realisation by American physicians of the need for measuring blood pressure in everyday practice [21].

18. Janeway T.C. A clinical study of hypertensive cardiovascular disease. *Archives of Internal Medicine* 1913; 12: 755-798.

19. It has too often been written in historical articles on the measurement of blood pressure that the manometer enabled the discovery of a new disease. This view is too narrow since one does not find a hidden treasure simply by owning a shovel, but rather by the desire to search, if necessary with the aid of a map...

20. Scholtz S.B. Notes on arterial hypertension from an American life insurance medicine viewpoint. *Proceedings of the 2nd congress of life insurance physicians.* Paris, May 18-21, 1939.

21. Despite Korotkoff's work in 1905 showing how diastolic blood pressure could be measured, most clinicians, insurance company physicians and teachers confined their measurements to the systolic blood pressure. It was only in 1917 that Fischer began to take an interest in the diastolic blood pressure. In 1921, as president of the association of life insurance medical directors of America, he convened a blood pressure committee which, the following year, recommended that the diastolic blood pressure be taken into account.

In 1911, Fischer addressed a letter to the Medical Directors Association which marked a turning point. In it, he explained that *"no doctor should practice medicine without a sphygmomanometer. The instrument is a reliable aid in the diagnostic procedure. The sphygmomanometer is indispensable for medical examination of life insurance applicants and the time is not far off when all companies will use it"* [22]. But what was the reasoning and what were the influences which led Fischer to make such a novel recommendation? He offers no explanation in his article and we were unable to find any bibliographic references to clarify this point. It must be realised that at the time Fischer recommended measuring blood pressure in all new life insurance applicants, there was no satisfactory publication on the prognosis related to blood pressure — it was still too early to speak of hypertension — and the only studies available were either purely descriptive or related to pathophysiology. Furthermore, a clear definition of normal blood pressure was still lacking. This highlights the originality of Fischer's approach. As early as 1907, Fischer began measuring the systolic blood pressure of life insurance applicants over the age of 40. He then went on to recruit physicians in cities of more than 100,000 inhabitants so that by 1913, 85% of all applicants to his company were having their blood pressure measured [20].

In 1909, Faught performed a survey of the experience of 32 of the major insurance companies. Ten of them did not measure blood pressure at all and the other 22 indicated that they recommended measurement of the systolic blood pressure when the age or the vascular status of the applicant suggested it was indicated [23]. At that time, the relationship between blood pressure and cardiovascular morbidity was still unknown. In 1910, Woley measured the blood pressure of a cohort of 1,000 subjects from 15 to 60 years old but this study was insufficient for insurance companies whose objective was to determine statistically an individual's life expectancy [24]. With no reliable studies to go on, the insurance companies had to produce their own statistics. Already well organised and well practised in the investigation of risk factors, it did not take them long to lay the foundations for the era of hypertension. Three years after his first written recommendation, that is in 1910, Fischer congratulated himself on his initiative: *"Today, the prediction has proven to be true. No up-to-date physician would deprive himself of the valuable diagnostic assistance of the sphygmomanometer, the usefulness of which has been emphasised by insurance company physicians. I have received hundreds of letters thanking me for recommending its use in insurance examinations and testifying to its usefulness in private practice"* [25]. It is noteworthy that Fischer refers to insurance company examinations and private practice but does not mention the hospital use of the sphygmomanometer which was still exceptional at this time.

22. Fischer. The diagnostic value of the sphygmomanometer in examinations for life insurance. *JAMA* Nov 14, 1914.

23. Faught. *New York Medical Journal.* July 1910. Quoted by S.B. Scholtz (20).

24. Woley H.P. Normal variations of the systolic pressure. *JAMA.* July 1910. Quoted by S.B Scholtz (20).

25. Quoted by Davis (4), p. 209.

In 1915, Mackenzie, working for the Prudential Life Insurance Company, had already acquired experience with 18,637 applicants [26]. Roger and Hunter of the New York Life Insurance Company measured the blood pressure of 62,000 insurance applicants. In 1922, Frost was able to report on the experience of the New York Metropolitan Life Insurance Company which totalised 500,000 examinations in over 8,000 policy holders [27]. The first large-scale surveys of blood pressure can thus be attributed to American insurance companies. Meanwhile, on the other side of the Atlantic, Vaquez expressed his surprise at how far behind the French insurance companies were: *"It is surprising to observe that in France life insurance company physicians are neglecting an examination which provides results that can have a considerable influence on their decisions"*, he commented [28]. Stévenin reiterated this reproach at the 2nd international congress of life insurance medicine (Paris 18-21 May 1939) when he denounced the failure of French physicians to keep up to date, stigmatised not only by their lack of technical skills but also by a lack of interest. *"There are still physicians who do not know how to perform this examination correctly"*, he deplored [29]. The American dominance in the area of insurance epidemiology can be accounted for essentially by the fact that in 1920, three quarters of all the life insurance policy holders in the world were in the United States! In 1941, some 9,000 American physicians were working for insurance companies [25]. From the 1920s up to the start of the Second World War, the statistics collected by insurance companies provided valuable information on the high prevalence of mild and moderate hypertension and its deleterious impact on affected individuals. It appears that Fischer was the first to establish a link between arterial pressure and mortality. In 1910, he refused to insure individuals whose systolic blood pressure was equal to or greater than 140 mmHg even though his own statistics only provided him with a follow-up of 2 years and 9 months [20]. During the same period, Scholtz reminds us, Mackenzie did not believe in this increased risk, despite the fact that mortality was three-fold higher amongst Fischer's applicants whose blood pressure was elevated (722 male subjects aged 20 to 60 years with a mean systolic pressure of 171 mmHg).

Insurance companies were also the instigators of studies into what was called 'isolated' hypertension, a form of hypertension too moderate to cause any clinical symptoms. Who else but the insurance company physician was sufficiently motivated to take an interest in this form of hypertension? In 1927, Pellissier once again emphasised the determinant role of the physician working for insurance companies *"Pure hypertension with a latent onset initially causes no symptoms. This is an important concept which warrants routine measurement of blood pressure to detect hypertension and to attempt to treat it at its very beginning. But it is not, generally speaking, in the hospital*

26. We will see later that this author came up with the idea of a prospective study which prefigured the Framingham study.

27. For details of these figures, see Henri Stévenin. La médecine d'assurance sur la vie. Facteurs biologiques, médicaux et sociaux de la mortalité et de la longévité. (Life insurance medicine. Biological medical and social factors of mortality and longevity). 1951. Masson, Paris. Op.cit.

28. Vaquez and Leconte. Passé, présent et avenir des hypertendus (The past, the present and the future of hypertensive individuals). *Paris Médical*. July 2nd, 1921.

29. To some extent, this is probably still true today.

ward that this initial phase is detected. Even in hospital out-patient departments, we usually only see these patients when they begin to have complaints: the latent phase is already over" [30].

30. Pellissier. *L'hypertension artérielle solitaire* (Isolated arterial hypertension). 1927, Paris .

THE NEED FOR STATISTICAL DATA:
A LESSON FROM THE INSURANCE COMPANIES

Although it was referred to as "latent" and "obscure", hypertension was nonetheless incredibly widespread and the problem of the boundary between normal and abnormal began to arise. In 1928, there was combined data on over one million subjects. In 1939, the 'Blood Pressure Study', based on statistical data from 15 or so insurance companies (totalling over 1,309,000 insurance policies!), confirmed the epidemic proportions of this new "disease". It is fair to say that physicians working for insurance companies made a much greater contribution than their other colleagues to the identification of this major risk factor. It took much longer for clinicians, cardiologists and general practitioners to recognise the importance of this finding. To quote Scholtz, they *"followed very slowly"* the teachings of the insurance companies [20]. In 1939, in his conclusion to the 2nd international congress of insurance company physicians, Dr Loéper remarked that *"If it is true, that certain statisticians know little about medicine, it is unfortunately even more true that most physicians know little or nothing about statistics. This is one of the great lessons to be learnt from the insurance companies"*.

The matter assumed such importance that shortly after the end of the Second World War, the American government became involved and in 1949, the National Health Service set up the National Heart Institute whose mission was to conduct an enquiry into asymptomatic cardiac conditions in a small town near Boston called Framingham. Another page in the history of hypertension was about to be written: that of therapeutic trials. The happy epilogue is that the relative success of treatment for hypertension has made it possible today for correctly treated and controlled hypertensive patients to benefit from the advantages of life insurance which they were formerly denied.

The Framingham enquiry
or epidemiology as a research tool

"In reality there are few if any individuals who die a natural death, led there by the inability to continue living. All are constantly exposed to causes of destruction against which they fight with a greater or lesser degree of success depending on their strength. [...] With regard to the human species, an understanding of the probability of dying is not only of the utmost importance for the physician, the administator and the economist, but it is also of the greatest importance for each of us. It may help us in the usual conduct of our lives to temper exaggerated fears or expectations; it may facilitate our submission to the severe laws of nature".

Antoine Augustin Cournot
Exposition de la théorie des chances et des probabilités
(On the theory of chance and probability).
1843

Statistics concerning questions of public health are nothing new. For centuries, births and deaths have been recorded in municipal and church registries. But these registries had nothing to do with epidemiology. In the 16th century, physicians became acquainted with large numbers for the study of the great epidemics such as the plague. But the counting of the victims was primarily intended for administrative purposes and cannot properly be called epidemiology in a modern sense. And when life expectancy was calculated for the very first time in the 17th century, the mathematical tools required (probability calculations) were only just beginning to be discovered. In the 18th century, the first quantitative evaluations of the efficacy of certain treatments (inoculation against smallpox, lemon against scurvy, etc) made their appearance and were the forerunners of early medical statistics. They aroused a certain amount of interest because at the time the authorities felt the need to control populations by influencing their health, longevity, birth rates and hygiene, thus introducing what Michel Foucault calls *"biopolitics"* [1]. The rise of urbanisation and the emergence of a working class created the need for quantifying certain pathological states potentially related to occupational or social factors. Figures became available on the prevalence of beggary, prostitution and alcoholism, laying the foundations for social epidemiology, in England first and then in France. It is noteworthy that death registries were set up at about this time.

1. Michel Foucault. *Résumé des Cours 1970-1982.* (Lecture summaries, 1970-1982. 1989. Julliard, Paris.

FROM HEALTH STATISTICS TO EPIDEMIOLOGY

These figures were used as snapshots of a society's state of health. But they were to adopt a new significance with the advent of the "numerate method". In the first half of the 19th century, the French physician Charles-Alexandre Louis began to cast a scientific, quantitative eye on the human body. He believed that a numerical approach would make it possible to quantify pathological states (which were later redefined by the anatomico-clinical method) with a view to evaluating how they evolved. This use of numbers was quite distinct from the health statistics of the 18th century. It was in fact a totally new way of looking at things, which Louis called "*la méthode numérique*" (the numerate method). With this innovation, Louis laid the foundations for modern medical statistics. Unfortunately his teachings were not received with much enthusiasm in his own country where voices were raised to denounce the "baneful interference of mathematics in medical science". By contrast, Louis' work was well received in England (by William Farr in particular) and in the United States [2].

Health statistics on pathological states could also be used to test hypotheses and to attempt to clarify causes of death. When blood pressure began to be measured at the end of the 19th century, heart disease was an unprecedented problem for the physician. Insurance companies, which were the first to ponder the prognostic significance of blood pressure recordings, could find no satisfactory studies concerning this point, and so they went about the task of gathering their own statistics. Their initiative was crowned with success and we recognise today that the concept of asymptomatic hypertension is truly their invention. The originality of their work stems not only from the fact that large numbers of subjects were included in the studies but also from the prospective nature of the investigations. Assumedly healthy individuals were recruited and examined for reasons unrelated to hypertension.

THE RAPID EXPANSION OF DEGENERATIVE AND CARDIOVASCULAR DISEASES BETWEEN THE TWO WORLD WARS

Between 1900 and 1930, life insurance companies were the only ones to take an interest in the epidemiology of hypertension. But when hospital and administrative death registries began to show an ever-increasing number of deaths due to degenerative diseases such as cancer and cardiovascular disorders, things began to change. Between 1930 and 1950, cardiovascular diseases gradually emerged as the primary cause of mortality. The beginnings of this increase can be traced back to the start of the 20th century. In the United States and in most European countries, the increase in longevity and the diminishing incidence of infectious diseases, particularly tuberculosis, began to change the statistics

2. For more information, see: Piquemal J. Succès et décadence de la méthode numérique en France à l'époque de Pierre-Charles-Alexandre Louis (The rise and fall of the numerate method in France at the time of Pierre-Charles-Alexandre Louis). In *Essais et leçons d'histoire de la médecine et de la biologie* (Essays and lessons on the history of medicine and biology). 1993. Presses Universitaires de France, Paris.

on mortality. Entries such as "tuberculosis" and "respiratory diseases" began to be overtaken by "haemorrhage" and "apoplexy". A statistical report in 1936, based on a registry of over 13,000 patients from a hospital in Paris, confirmed this tendency. The report stated that the mortality due to cardiovascular diseases had increased significantly in the past 30 years. The registry classified cardiovascular disorders into 3 groups: functional disturbances, organic cardiac disease, and vessel disease. The third group included entries such as aortitis, angina pectoris, obliterating arteritis, Raynaud's syndrome, diseases of the veins and arterial hypertension. This last group was broken down into mild, moderate or severe. Interestingly, it was the hypertension group that was the largest [3].

Despite the growing evidence, the health authorities did not devote significant resources to cardiovascular medicine between the two world wars. During this period, cancer was the centre of attention and consumed most of the available resources [4]. There were, however, a few longitudinal studies begun in the 1920s, and the cardiologist Sir James Mackenzie attempted to identify what he called the *"beginnings of illness"* by performing an epidemiological study in Scotland. His premature death in 1925 left this work unfinished, but his colleague Paul Dudley White pursued the idea and exported it to Boston. A major task lay ahead.

During the 1939-1945 war, cardiovascular diseases did not receive a high priority rating from the health authorities in the United States because great demands were being made on epidemiologists by the American army whose soldiers where paying a heavy tribute to hepatitis, malaria and yellow fever [5]. But American medicine did not remain behind in cardiovascular research for very long.

FRAMINGHAM: FROM OBSERVATION TO UNDERSTANDING

In 1949, cardiovascular disease accounted for half the deaths recorded in the United States [6]. During the 1950s, one male in three appeared to develop cardiovascular disease before reaching the age of 60 [7]. The observed decline in infant mortality was having little effect on the life expectancy of individuals over the age of 45 in whom degenerative diseases were taking a heavy toll. At that time, myocardial infarction was a major cause of death as there was no effective treatments and heart attack victims usually died before reaching hospital [8].

In order to clarify the situation in a context where some still doubted that half of all mortality could be of cardiovascular origin, the National Heart Institute of the United States Public Health Service decided, in October 1947, to undertake a vast epidemiological study in the city of Framingham, Massachusetts.

3. Lian C., Cahana J. La fréquence croissante de la morbidité et de la mortalité dues aux affections cardiovasculaires (The increasing frequency of morbidity and mortality due to cardiovascular disease). *La Presse médicale*, 1936. N°52, pp. 1061-1062.

4. See Pinell P. *Naissance d'un fléau: histoire de la lutte contre le cancer en France, 1890-1940* (The emergence of an epidemic: history of the fight against cancer in France). 1992; Métailié, Paris.

5. For the history of American epidemiology, see Susser M. Epidemiology in the United States after World War II: the evolution of techniques. *Epidemiologic Reviews*, 1985; 7:147-177.

6. Kannel W. Contribution of the Framingham Study to preventive cardiology. *JACC*, 1990; 15:206-211.

7. Kannel W. Contribution of the Framingham Study to the conquest of coronary artery disease. *Am J Cardiol* 1988; 1109-1112.

8. Because many patients died at home during this period, it is difficult to interpret the medical literature which is based essentially on hospital statistics. It is surprising to read today how many authors emphasised the relative rareness of myocardial infarction diagnosed in hospital during the period 1920 -1940.

Initially directed by Thomas Dawber [9], the study came under the control of the National Heart Institute, newly created on July 1, 1949. The objective of the study was to survey for 20 years the population of 28,000 inhabitants of the city of Framingham, considered to be representative of the American urban way of life, for the onset of events related to "arteriosclerotic heart disease". This initial formulation was later changed to "ischaemic heart disease" for reasons of classification and indexing.

The implementation of this wide-scale prospective approach was an entirely new initiative. Never before had such data been collected. An enquiry of this type was needed because pre-war epidemiological enquiries had been designed not for long-term degenerative diseases but essentially for infectious diseases. Cardiovascular disorders posed different problems. Their onset could not be determined with accuracy, there was no incubation period and there did not appear to be a single causative agent as with infectious diseases [10].

The first subjects to enter the study were examined in September 1948. Four years later, 5,209 men and women from 30 to 62 years old had been recruited to the survey which was to become a reference in modern epidemiology [11]. The subjects had no evidence of cardiovascular disease and had all accepted to undergo a medical examination every two years. Although the number of subjects recruited was very large it was, however, slightly lower than the projected figure of 6,000 subjects. Other volunteers were recruited subsequently.

From a practical standpoint, the initial aim was to identify differences between individuals who developed cardiovascular disease and those who did not. Since the microscope, the scalpel and biochemical analyses had, for the past century, failed to elucidate artherosclreoris, apoplexy and coronary artery disease, a new approach was needed: that of prospective epidemiology. The advent of this new field just after the Second World War marked a conceptual turning point. The aim was no longer simply to observe, but also to understand. "Descriptive" epidemiology was becoming "deductive" epidemiology. This evolution was apparent not only in the Framingham enquiry but in all the epidemiology literature of the time and was further reinforced by the emergence of young epidemiology societies and the introduction of specific university courses. It was from the impetus of what has been called the "epidemiologic transition" (that is a decline in infection-related deaths and a rise in degenerative diseases) that the Framingham enquiry derived its justification. New methodological tools were making their appearance. The cross-sectional field surveys used in the 1920s and 1930s were now considered inadequate and prospective surveys of large cohorts to determine disease incidence appeared. As stated earlier, this was a new idea and no mention of it can be found in books on epidemiology published at the time when the Framingham study was

9. And then by William Kannel from 1966 onwards.

10. Dawber T., Kannel W. The epidemiology of coronary heart disease. The Framingham Enquiry. *Proceedings of the Society of Medicine.* 1962; 55: 265-271.

11. The Framingham Study. *DHEW Publication* (NIH). 74-478. Dec. 1973.

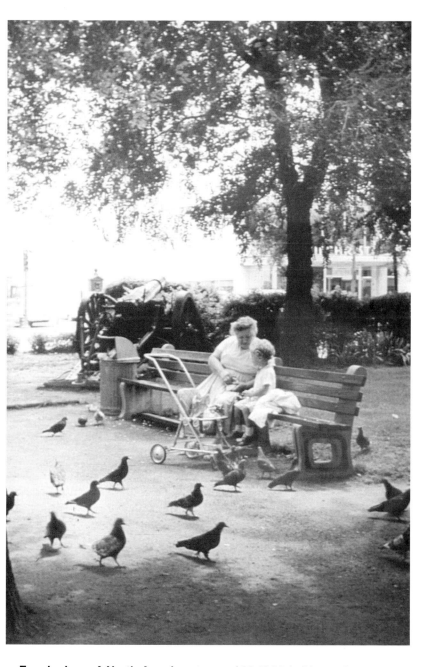

Framingham: A North-American town of 28,000 inhabitants became an international reference.

The first major prospective study on vascular risk factors began in Framingham in 1947. For 20 years, epidemiologists searching for the causes of cardiovascular death, had their eyes focused on this American town of 28,000 inhabitants considered to be representative of the American urban way of life. Success lay at the end of the road and 20 years after its implementation, the Framingham enquiry had become a model for post-war epidemiology.

beginning. This silence continued for several years and the methodological theory used in the Framingham study (notably the study of sociological variables) found its way into the literature only in the early 1960s [5]. By this time, other multivariate analyses in cardiovascular epidemiology were flourishing, aided by the availability of new computers capable of performing thousands of elementary operations in a few seconds. It had now become easier to apply the multivariate analytical strategies required to take into account causal relationships and eliminate confounding variables. The widespread use of a special technique of multivariate analysis, linear regression, was further facilitated by the possibility of categorising continuous variables into discreet variables in regression equations. This technique of dummy variables was introduced around 1957.

THE IDENTIFICATION OF RISK FACTORS

When the Framingham enquiry began, it was thought that a limited number of atherogenic factors would be found. For this reason, smoking was not initially taken into account. In fact the number of factors proved to be much greater than initially anticipated. As time went by, new variables were measured and additional lifestyle factors were taken into account. Assays for serum cholesterol became possible in October 1950. As with any pioneering enquiry, the aims and methods of the study evolved and grew as new data was collected. Thus, the idea of cardiovascular risk factors, still a vague concept in 1948, gradually became clearer. Concomitantly, methodological problems arose but the very strength of the study, i.e. its long duration, made it possible to avoid the pitfalls. According to Daniel Schwartz (1981), "*risk is determined by our ignorance and by chance. The role of the epidemiologist is to reduce our ignorance as much as possible with the ultimate aim of coming as close as possible (generally without reaching it) to the moment where risk is determined by chance alone*" [12].

In the Framingham study, ignorance was certainly present, since the factors underlying vascular risks had not yet been identified. Chance, as always in statistics, remained an inevitable component but it had now been brought under control as far as possible by probability calculations. The 1950s saw the end of an era during which investigators hesitated or remained discreetly silent in the face of two different concepts. Was hypertension a disease, and in this case, was there a distinct boundary between patients and healthy individuals? Or was the reality more complex? Did it involve several levels of severity or different causes? Fischer's uncertainty about the level above which an individual could be considered as hypertensive testified to these difficulties as far back as 1914. In a general review published in 1931 in the *JAMA*, David Riesman expressed the perplexity he experienced

12. Cited by A. Fagot-Largeault. Présent et futur de l'épidémiologie (The present and future of epidemiology). *Colloque INSERM*, 1988; 159: 63-72.

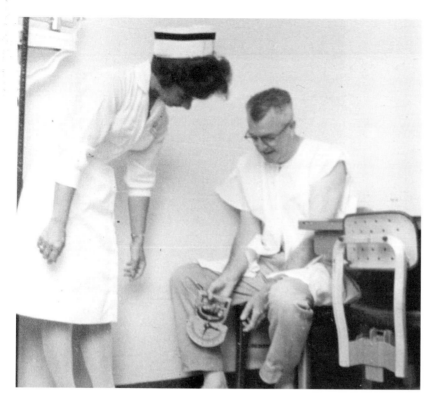

Framingham: a broad view to validate the concept of a multifactorial disease

The initial parameters chosen for the Framingham study were both broad and incomplete since, in 1947, not only were cardio-vascular risk factors poorly known, but they were also poorly understood. Smoking was not initially included. In contrast, spirometric or dynamometric data were recorded (it may be noted in passing that certain insurance companies were already using spirometry at the end of the 19th century). The scales visible in the top photograph quickly proved their worth by demonstrating that obesity was a cardiovascular risk factor (a fact which doctors studying mortality due to cerebral apoplexy had already suggested half a century earlier). Today the investigators, satisfied that they have achieved the initial objectives of identifying vascular risk factors, are turning their attention to the study of age-related disorders such as osteoporosis and cancer.

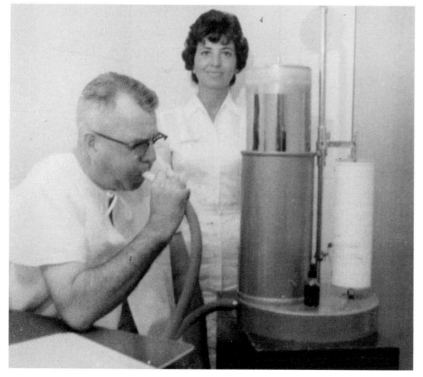

The Framingham enquiry: epidemiology overtakes clinical and laboratory medicine

In 1948, the factors responsible for atherogenesis had not been identified and the methodology for prospective studies had not been definitively established. By collecting an enormous number of data and by performing a long-term statistical analysis (top) the Framingham enquiry succeeded in identifying the factors related to cardiovascular mortality and morbidity thus leading to the concept of a multifactorial disease (bottom left). Contrary to what is suggested in the bottom right photograph, the microscope was of little assistance in helping to understand cardiovascular mortality (bottom right). In effect, the epidemiological methods applied to infectious diseases were inappropriate for the study of the causes of degenerative disorders.

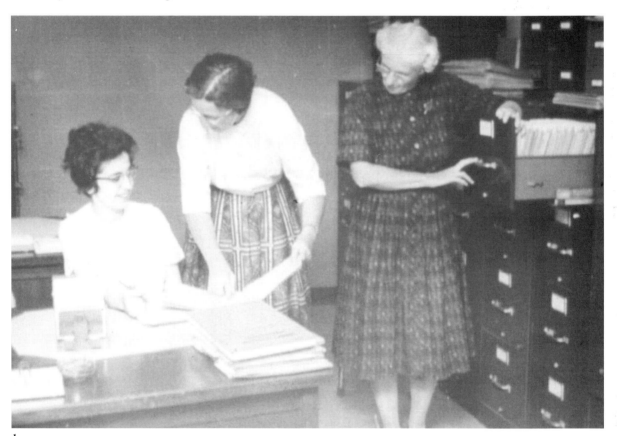

1

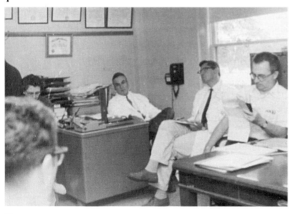

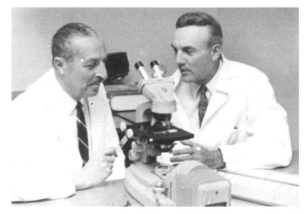

2

3

as a clinician with the emerging concept of risk factors [13]. He reported the results obtained from several insurance companies but expressed surprise at the fact that he knew patients whose longevity contrasted with an elevated blood pressure [14]. The controversy between Platt and Pickering came to an end in the 1950s with the outcome being in favour of the latter [15]. It was now recognised that there were not two populations, as Platt had suggested, but only one in which blood pressure, like many other biological variables, was normally distributed (Gaussian curve).

After twenty years of follow-up, the National Heart Institute announced that the Framingham study had achieved its initial objectives in identifying the major vascular risk factors. After some years of deliberation, the decision was made to pursue the enquiry but to reformulate its aims and to extend it beyond the cardiovascular horizon.

In a quarter of a century, the Framingham study had identified and documented the major risk factors for cardiovascular disease and atheroma. The involvement, or responsibility of hereditary factors, lifestyle, serum lipid levels, blood pressure levels, blood sugar and fibrinogen were all revealed. Amongst the lifestyle factors, an accusing finger was pointed at the excessive intake of calories, fat and salt, a sedentary lifestyle, obesity and smoking. Alcohol was given a "suspended sentence" for good conduct because consumed in moderation, it was associated with a low incidence of cardiovascular events. Coffee was practically acquitted [16]. Spirometric measurement of vital capacity (performed by insurance companies as far back as the turn of this century) was shown to be a good independent predictor of cardiovascular mortality, though this method never acquired the popularity of blood pressure measurement. A typical behavioral profile of the potential cardiovascular victim was even defined: the candidate was a person with hostile, time-urgent, competitive behaviour (so-called Type A). The enquiry, which left no avenue unexplored, was even able to show that men married to highly-educated women who worked outside the home were at increased risk! [17].

After showing an increase for many years, to reach almost epidemic proportions in the 1960s, the incidence of cardiovascular disease began to decline. This decline coincided with the increasing sophistication of medical care and a concerted effort to reduce risk factors. In the United States, changes in eating habits, the reduction in smoking, and the control of serum cholesterol and blood pressure levels are paying dividends today. For the enthusiasts, this decline proved the success of the Framingham enquiry which was the first to encourage the control of risk factors [18]. It prompted physicians to fight smoking in the 1960s, hypertension in the 1970s and cholesterol in the 1980s. In other words, Framingham was an example of epidemiology leading to the treatment of risk factors by modifying lifestyle and by drug therapy.

13. A variable is defined as a risk factor for an event if its value is proportional to the probability of onset of that event.

14. Riesman D. High blood pressure and longevity. *JAMA* 1931; 96: 1105-1111.

15. According to Platt, there were two genetically determined populations. The first was a normotensive population whose blood pressure rose gradually with age. The second consisted of hypertensive individuals whose blood pressure could rise with age to levels likely to cause complications. Platt R. The nature of essential hypertension. *Lancet* 1959; 2: 55.

16. Kannel W.B. Coffee, cocktails and coronary candidates (editorial) *N Engl J Med* 1977; 297: 443-444.

17. Eaker E.D., Haynes S.G., Feinleb M. Spouse behavior and coronary heart disease in man: prospective results from the Framingham Heart Study. Eaker E.D., Haynes S.G., Feinleb M. Modifications of risks in type A husbands according to the social and psychological status of their wives. *Am J Epidemiol* 1983; 117: 23-41. (But what can medicine can do about this...?)

18. Although nothing had been proved in 1962. Dawber T., Kannel W. The epidemiology of coronary heart disease. The Framingham Enquiry. *Proceedings of the Society of Medicine.* 1962; 55: 265-271.

THE "CAUSES" OF CARDIOVASCULAR RISK:
MORE THAN WAS BARGAINED FOR

Another achievement of the Framingham enquiry was to have validated the concept of a multifactorial disease. The victory of Pasteur's conceptions in the 19th century had confined investigations into the causes of infectious disease to tracking down the microorganism responsible. This monofactorial perspective dominated the thinking on causality for many years. Thus, in the pursuit of the causes of infectious diseases, criteria of causality called "Koch's postulates" were defined [19]. Hypertension did not conform to this conception and one of the challenges for the Framingham investigators was to call into question Koch's postulates. They got more than they bargained for, but a certain ambivalence remained as to whether certain risk factors represented what was called causes or determinants of hypertension. The interactions between blood pressure and environmental factors are so complex that investigations into causality tend to get lost in conjecture.

With the availability of new sophisticated investigational tools such as ultrasound, the Framingham study began to explore new areas such as the prognostic significance of myocardial hypertrophy, changes in contractility and the ejection fraction. The list of biochemical assays grew longer as new laboratory techniques became available. The validity of portable blood pressure recorders was studied. As the population of the city grew older, Framingham cast its epidemiological eye on horizons beyond cardiovascular disease. Today the enquiry has turned its attention to senile dementia, osteoporosis, emphysema and degenerative joint disease. This extension may be interpreted as the rebirth of the enquiry but it may also be a sign that we are perhaps in the process of reaching the methodological limits of the Framingham enquiry.

The fact remains that the Framingham study has become the symbol of the victory of epidemiology which has proven capable of elucidating the causes of chronic disorders and tracking down the *"beginnings of illness"* that James MacKenzie pursued in the 1920s. Framingham constitutes a model for cohort studies of which it has inspired many others. By inaugurating the era of long-term population surveys, it has had a profound impact on the history of epidemiology, to such an extent that it has become the standard-bearer of the field. In fact, we no longer even say "the Framingham study" but just simply "Framingham". What was once the name of a town has now become the name of a study.

19. Koch considered that to prove a causal relationship between a microorganism and a disease, it had to be established that:
1) the microorganism was always present in subjects with the disease;
2) the microorganism was never present in patients without the disease;
3) the microorganism could be recovered from an infected subject, grown in pure culture and shown to reproduce the disease when innoculated into a healthy subject. Cited by A. Fagot-Largeault. Approches médicales de la causalité dans les systèmes complexes (A medical approach to causality in complex systems). *Arch Int Physiol Biochim* 1986; 94: C85-94. See also Anne Fagot-Largeault. *Les causes de la mort, histoire naturelle et facteurs de risque* (The causes of death, natural history and risk factors). 1989; Vrin, Paris.

3
UNDERSTANDING HYPERTENSION

Too many questions and an unclassifiable entity

"So many foolish things have been said and written about blood pressure that I am obliged to draw attention to our extreme ignorance as to the causes and consequences of an elevated blood pressure".

Sir James MacKenzie
1926

When Stephen Hales connected a cannula to the artery of a mare in 1733, he made the very first experimental measurement of the *"force of the blood"* which up to that time had only been the object of theoretical speculation. Subsequently, physiologists conceived devices for studying animals, and later man, which allowed clinicians such as Basch and Potain to introduce the measurement of blood pressure into hospital practice at the end of the 19th century. The values thus recorded raised many questions: How is blood pressure regulated? What does an elevated reading signify? Is hypertension a disease? And if so, what is it due to?

COMPLEMENTARY AND CONFLICTING THEORIES

The history of our understanding of blood pressure regulation and of the recognition of secondary forms of hypertension is characterised above all by its complexity. For over a hundred years, generations of physiologists and clinicians have attempted to elucidate these problems. Along the way, some have got lost and some have encountered success. The difficulties they had to face were immense and even today many questions regarding hypertension have still not been unequivocally answered. For example, clinicians view Conn's syndrome as a disease while epidemiologists define essential hypertension as a risk factor. As for biologists and geneticists, they emphasise the diversity of situations that come under the heading "arterial hypertension".

In fact, researchers were faced with two questions: the pathophysiology underlying blood pressure elevation on the one hand, and its pathological significance on the other. These were two difficult and quite distinct questions. And so it was on quite shaky ground that numerous theories of the regulation of normal and abnormal blood pressure attempted to elucidate the causes of blood pressure elevation. As the years passed, different theories came into fashion. At the very beginning of the 20th century, adrenal gland disorders were commonly believed to be the main, if not the only cause of hypertension. At other times, kidney disorders or salt inbalance were the most popular candidates. Some investigators suggested the existence of endocrine mechanisms, others preferred to study vasomotor phenomena while others still favoured a renal or biochemical origin. The relative importance of these theories varied in a somewhat haphazard and non-chronological fashion. The different approaches overlapped, interacted or contradicted each other in a climate of confusion that was understandable given the multifactorial and elusive nature of hypertension. In the face of these difficulties, clinicians were tempted to give up the search and the concept of essential hypertension emerged quite early, suggested in particular by Mahomed and Allbutt. Back in 1915, Allbutt suggested grouping blood pressure elevations under the term "hyperpiesia". He defined this term as *a disease in which blood pressure rises abnormally in middle life* [1].

1. Allbutt T.C. Diseases of the arteries including angina pectoris; 1915. Macmillan, London.

HYPERTENSION: A SYMPTOM, A REACTION OR A DISEASE?

The first clinicians to take an interest in blood pressure levels had to answer a crucial question: is high blood pressure the cause or the consequence of the deterioration of the cardiovascular or renal system?

This question, a key issue in the history of hypertension as a disease, divided two schools of thought for at least 20 years. The first believed in the anatomico-clinical method while the second put their faith in experimental medicine. The former based their reasoning on the anatomical lesions they observed. The latter relied on pathophysiological considerations (which in the case of arterial pressure linked the heart, the vessels and the kidneys in a succession of events). The "anatomists" recruited their subjects in the morgues, and sought the truth by exploring corpses with their scalpels. The "experimentalists" found their subjects in the laboratory and worked with dogs connected to manometers. With such opposing views, it is not surprising that the two schools had little respect for one another until the first half of the 20th century. They had totally different ideas about the origin of diseases and they were in total disagreement over the problem of the causes and consequences of disease. Claude Bernard denounced these differences of opinion. *"The anatomopathologists claim to demonstrate that anatomical alterations are always the primary cause of disease. I do not believe this. On the contrary, it is my belief that very often pathological alterations are the consequence or the result of disease rather than the cause"* [2].

2. Bernard C. cited by Vaquez in: *La pression moyenne de l'homme à l'état normal et pathologique* (Mean pressure in man in health and disease).1936, Paris.

Concepts of arterial hypertension: the early pre-eminence of morbid anatomy

The anatomico-clinical method, i.e. the correlation between clinical signs during life with organ changes observed at autopsy, revolutionised medical thinking in the 19th century. For many years its influence created confusion between hypertension and arteriosclerosis, both conceptually and therapeutically. In a widely cited work, Charcot, in 1868, identified cerebral micro-aneurysms as the determinant cause of cerebral haemorrhage (J.M. Charcot, *Archives de Physiologie Normale et Pathologique* I, 1868; pp. 110,643,725). With the invention of the sphygmomanometer and the advent of the experimental and epidemiological approaches to hypertension, the microscope was forgotten and replaced by the concept of risk factors and regulation of blood pressure.

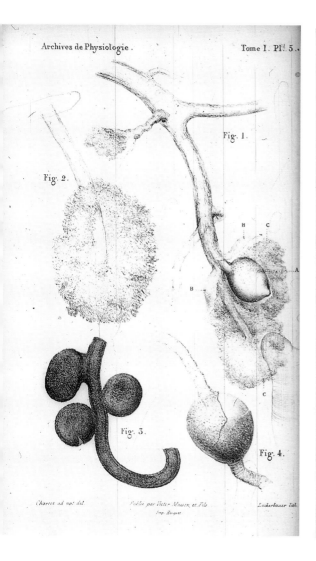

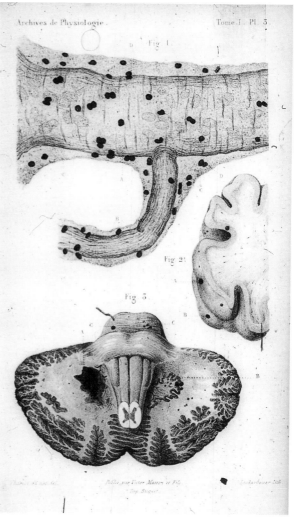

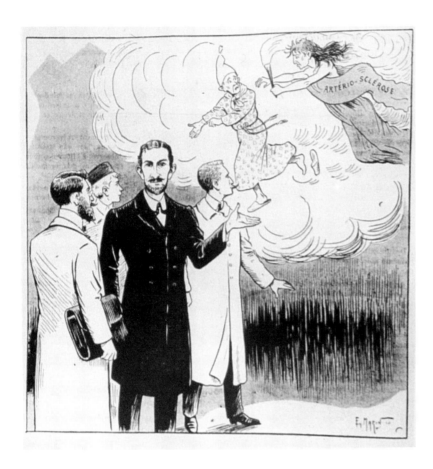

"Arteriosclerosis pursuing humanity"

It had been known since the 18th century that with increasing age the blood vessels became "ossified" and the anatomist's scalpel made an unmistakable sound as it crunched through the frail remnants of "senile arteries". In the 19th century, haunted by "degenerations" of all sorts, there was a mortal fear of arteriosclerosis which was considered by some to be the "scourge" of humanity. It was in this context, in the middle of the 19th century, that life insurance company physicians learned to recognise this vascular alteration clinically by using the sphygmometer even before the invention of the sphygmomanometer. The caption on the poster says: «Notice, Gentlemen, the spectre of arteriosclerosis pursuing humanity».

In 1902, Potain rejected the possibility that an elevated pressure could cause hypertrophy of the heart, sclerosis of the vessels and albuminuria, whereas Basch, and later Huchard were of a different opinion. Prospective epidemiology was to clarify the situation.

In the opinion of some, the anatomical abnormalities (arterial and renal sclerosis had been known since the early 19th century) were the cause of hypertension. But then how could one explain these curious silent and obscure forms of hypertension which insurance company physicians were discovering in asymptomatic patients in whom albuminuria was not always present? Depending on the clinical expression of blood pressure elevation (severe and symptomatic or moderate and silent), physicians hesitated between several denominations: "hypertension-symptom", "hypertension-syndrome" and "hypertension-disease"[3]. The time factor was the key in determining "hypertension disease". It was crucial for insurance company physicians, who accused hypertension of reducing life expectancy, and it was crucial for Nature to create anatomical lesions. The realisation of the importance of the time factor was a key element in the epistemology of hypertension. The conflict between the "anatomists" and the "experimentalists" arose because the time factor had been overlooked. Leriche clearly explained this in his *Basis of physiological surgery*[4].

Dumas explained that *"hypertension is a disorder affecting the entire arterial system in which elevated blood pressure is the major symptom and the only one in the early phase. Later multiple visceral symptoms become apparent"*[5]. If the anatomo-pathologist intervened too early, he saw nothing because the lesion had not yet had time to develop, whereas at this stage the physiologist already recognised "a disease". Initially viewed as a "symptom" when blood pressure was simply considered to reflect a measurement, hypertension became a disorder that Laubry in 1930 and Dumas in 1939 described as *"a disease in its own right"*[6].

In 1910, Gallavardin published a book on blood pressure in clinical medicine, its measurement and semiological value. In this book, blood pressure continued to be intrepreted within the framework of known diseases and was not really considered as a new disease entity. Ten years later, in the preface to the 2nd edition of his book (1920), Gallavardin again stated that *"sphygmomanometry is to chronic diseases what the thermometer is to acute diseases"*[7]. However, he did develop a chapter on the concept of *"isolated hypertension"* based on *"mechanical and humoral theories"*. In this chapter he stated that *"it is necessary to go one step beyond a simple inventory of blood pressure changes in various diseases"*, as Potain had done in his 1902 publication where he considered blood pressure simply as a reflection of infectious, renal or cardiovascular disorders.

3. Dumas A., in: *La maladie hypertensive* (Hypertensive disease). 1939, Paris (p. 13).

4. Leriche R. *Bases de la chirurgie physiologique; Essai sur la vie végétative des tissus.*(Basis of physiological surgery; an essay on the vegetative life of tissues). 1933. Masson , Paris.

5. Potain believed that blood pressure simply reflected general health. It was low in typhoid fever, elevated in renal disease and simply followed the state of the body. In contrast, Basch wondered very early if a rise in blood pressure could not cause disease *per se*.

6. *"Isolated elevation of blood pressure reflects a profound and primary circulatory disturbance. Diagnosed among other cardiovascular or visceral alterations, the importance or autonomy of hypertension is such that these other alterations may be considered to be under its dependence. It is no longer a chance finding, nor the abnormal result of measurement. It is a disease in its own right and should be studied as such".*
Laubry C. in: *Nouveau traité de pathologie interne* (New treatise on internal medicine). 1930. vol. III. Maladies des vaisseaux (Blood vessel diseases). p. 845.
"Chronic progressive hypertension is a disease which, from its very beginnings, affects the entire arterial system [...]. This is essential hypertension, a term which means that hypertension is not simply a symptom but a disease in its own right". Dumas A. *ibid.* p. 13.

7. Gallavardin L. *La Tension artérielle en clinique. Sa mesure, sa valeur sémiologique* (Blood pressure in clinical medicine, its measurement and semiological value). 1920, Masson, Paris. p. 233.

The conceptual vagueness surrounding the significance of hypertension as a "symptom" or a "disease" is well illustrated by attempts to single out a "mirror-image" disease — arterial hypotension. In 1931, Giraud published a book on arterial hypotension in chronic diseases and described "*a symptom which cannot easily be classified as primary or secondary*" [8]. This book reported on the work of the 20th French congress of medicine (Society of French Physicians, Montpellier, October 15-17, 1929). In 1936, Vaquez refuted the reality of hypotension as a disease. He wrote "*Hypotension as a disease was the object of discussion during a congress held in Montpellier. Much effort was devoted to proving the reality of this entity. It appears that these efforts have not been successful and the only observation of real interest was a study presented by an American author in which hypotension, rather than being a threat, was in fact shown to be a blessing and a guarantee of long life. What a strange disease!*" [9].

The emergence of the concept that hypertension was a disease was not a simple matter. It was envisioned by Gallavardin under the term "*permanent arterial hypertension*" defined as "*a circulatory disorder which was not described in medical treatises ten or twenty years ago and which is, in reality, the underlying cause of a number of pathological states*". Hypertension was still trying to find its rightful place in disease classification and Gallavardin remarked that "*rather than being a disease in the restrictive sense, hypertension is a mode of reaction of the sick individual, and it has infinitely vaster implications*".

A "CHEMICAL FAULT"

Forty years after Gallavardin, the contribution of life insurance companies, which had succeeded in relating statistically elevated blood pressure and life expectancy, did not put an end to the debate on the classification of hypertension. Many physicians continued to stress the difficulty of describing and classifying this "disease". Discouraged by all these hesitations, George Pickering recognised that the concept of arterial hypertension as a specific entity was not consistent with the observed facts and should be reconsidered [10]. In effect, the anatomico-clinical approach was of little use when it came to hypertension. Although in earlier times, it had been dominant in designating "Bright's disease", "arteriosclerosis" and then "pre-sclerosis" (Huchard), this approach had reached its limits in many situations of elevated blood pressure. This led Pickering to state that it was pointless to continue searching for a clear-cut boundary between normal and abnormal blood pressure [11].

But history continued to confuse the issue because that same year, 1955, Conn discovered primary aldosteronism, which was based of course on an anatomical criterion (a tumour) and in which the pathologic abnormality was clearly visible. And so, attention was turned to the possibility that hypertension might be related to a

8. Giraud G. *L'hypotension artérielle dans les maladies chroniques* (Arterial hypotension in chronic diseases). Paris 1931.

9. Vaquez in: *La pression moyenne, de l'homme à l'état normal et pathologique* (Mean blood pressure in health and disease) 1936, Paris. p. 112.

10. Pickering G. The concept of essential hypertension. *Ann Int Med* 1955, 43: 1153-1160.

11. For more on this important point, see chapter 5 — The question of norms.

"chemical fault", a concept which can in fact be traced back to over a century earlier [12]. Its history is not linear and some of its essential features will be discussed with the discovery of the renin-angiotensin system, pheochromocytoma and Conn's syndrome.

12. The term "chemical fault" was used by G. Pickering in his book *Hypertension, causes, consequences and management.* 1970. Churchill, London.

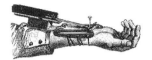

The discovery of the renin-angiotensin system

"It is always dangerous to rest in a narrow pathology; and I believe that to be a narrow pathology which is satisfied with what you now see before me on this table. In this glass you see a much hypertrophied heart, and a very contracted kidney. This specimen is classical. It was, I believe, put up under Dr. Bright's own direction, and with a view of showing that the wasting of the kidney is the cause of the thickening of the heart. I cannot but look upon it with veneration, but not with conviction. I think, with all deference to so great an authority, that the systemic capillaries, and, had it been possible, the entire man, should have been included in this vase, together with the heart and the kidneys; and then we should have had, I believe, a truer view of the causation of the cardiac hypertrophy, and of the disease of the kidney".

William Gull
Clinical lecture on chronic Bright's disease with contracted kidney
(arteriocapillary sclerosis).
Brit Med J 1872, 2: 707-709.

Back in the 17th and 18th centuries, the anatomists had already remarked the dilatation and hypertrophy of the heart, particularly when valve disease was present. But the credit for observing the existence of left ventricular hypertrophy in certain renal disorders goes to Richard Bright.

RICHARD BRIGHT: A "FUNCTIONAL" CONCEPTION OF MORBID ANATOMY

In London in 1827, Richard Bright, a physician at Guy's Hospital published the first volume of his famous *Reports of medical cases*. The reports contained a detailed collection of the histories and observations of large numbers of Bright's patients followed by a description of autopsy findings. Bright was following the innovative example of the Paris School (Bichat, Corvisart and Laënnec) who founded the anatomico-clinical method some twenty years earlier in the early 19th century. This revolution in medical thinking was the guiding influence for Bright's undertaking and he very quickly realised *"the importance of that information which our profession derives from the study of the Morbid Anatomy"*. The French had already acquired considerable knowledge of lung diseases. Bright chose to study dropsies and kidney diseases, about which little was known in the first half of the 19th century. Bright justified his approach in the following words: "*To connect accurate and faithful observation after death with symptoms displayed during life, must be in some degree to forward the objects of our noble art: and the more extensive the observation, and the more close the connexion which can be traced, the more likely we are to discover the real analogy and dependence which exists, both between functional and organic disease, and between these, and the external symptoms which are alone submitted to our investigation during life*" [1]. Although Bright did not invent the method, he used it in a novel manner. In 1827, he had already collected 30 cases of patients suffering from "*anasarca and ascites with coagulable urine*" [2]. He was the first to propose an anatomical classification of kidney diseases.

Encouraged by his peers, Bright pursued the immense task he had set himself. In 1831, he published 310 anatomico-clinical cases in the second volume of Medical Reports. According to Bright, the lesions of the different organs of the body were determined by three types of morbid conditions: "*inflammation, pressure and irritation*". The term "pressure" had never before been used in medical terminology and Bright confessed to the hesitation that the word had caused him: "*I have likewise adopted "pressure" as the generic term of the second section, but not without hesitation; for in many of the cases which it includes, the influence of pressure is by no means capable of demonstration, and it probably does not exist. The term disruption of the circulation or disruption of cerebral influence would no doubt be more appropriate*" [3]. In fact, by the term "pressure", Bright was referring to all of the neurological aspects associated with cerebral vascular accidents which he designated as "*effects of cerebral pressure resulting from cerebral swelling and distension, cerebral haemorrhage, cerebral tumours or hydrocephalus*". The term "*pressure*" was therefore not a premonition of the future concept of blood pressure, and even less so of hypertensive disease as conceived by Basch and Potain at the end of the 19th century. Bright's remarks in 1831 have no direct relationship to the history of blood pressure but they show that he was aware of the concept of function and that he was no longer simply looking for anatomical alterations. He was driven by a modern and dynamic conception which led him to study the interrelationships between organs. Although he did not use the term physiology or pathophysiology, Bright wondered about the time sequence of anatomical alterations of organs and their function. Like Claude Bernard in the mid 19th century and Leriche in the early 20th century, Bright stated: "*I believe that functional disease in this, as in most other cases, precedes the structural change*" [4]. This remark revealed great foresight and was to assume particular relevance in 1836 when Bright published a very important work for the history of hypertensive disease.

1. Bright R. *Reports of medical cases.* 1827. Preface p. VII. For more on the anatomico-clinical method and the Paris School, which attracted many students from Britain, see E.H. Ackerknecht. *La Médecine hospitalière à Paris* (Hospital medicine in Paris). 1986. Payot, Paris.

2. Out of a total of 90 cases which also included liver and lung diseases and febrile intestinal manifestations.

3. R. Bright. *Reports of medical cases selected with a view of illustrating plates.* 1831, vol. 2, preface p. VIII.

4. Bright R. *Reports of medical cases.* 1827. Preface p. X.

BRIGHT AND GULL: The unexplained observation of a relationship between renal alterations and cardiac enlargement, or the limits of morbid anatomy.

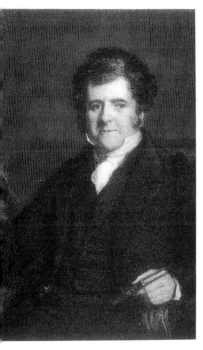

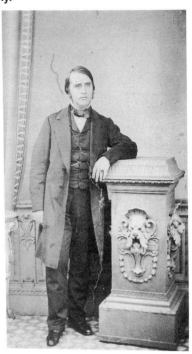

The British pathologist Richard Bright (1789-1858) (left) was the first to emphasise, in 1836, the presence of left ventricular hypertrophy in patients who died of renal failure with albuminuria. However, contrary to what is sometimes believed, Bright did not clearly suggest that raised blood pressure was the underlying factor for the pathological processes affecting the heart and the kidneys.

William Gull (right), Bright's successor at Guy's hospital, was not convinced by Brights hypothesis. He did not believe that the renal atrophy was directly responsible for the cardiac enlargement, and in 1872 he put forward the idea that an alteration of the *«systemic capillaries»* was the true common denominator.

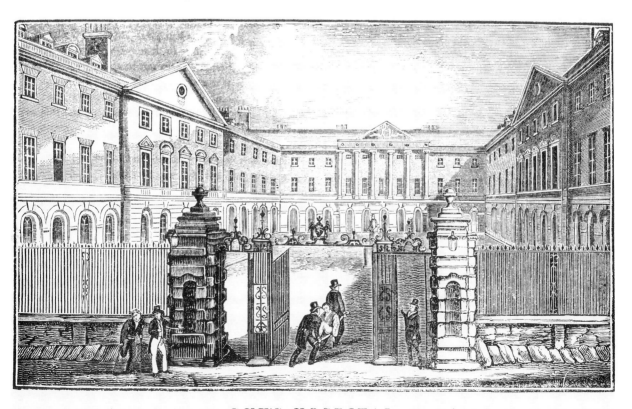

GUY'S HOSPITAL.

In his *"Tabular view of the morbid appearances in 100 cases connected with albuminous urine"*, Bright gave a detailed description of the anatomico-clinical aspects of the victims of renal disease. He verified that in a large proportion of the victims, albuminuria was present before death and he attended each autopsy personally. For each case, Bright recorded not only the cause of death but an anatomical description of the kidneys and the state of various other organs such as the pleura, the lung, pericardium, heart, abdominal cavity, peritoneum, liver, intestine, stomach, spleen, pancreas, aorta, brain, uterus and gall bladder. After remarking that there were severe alterations in the circulatory and respiratory systems as well as the serous membranes, Bright noted that the *"changes in the state of the heart are most noteworthy"*. Such changes were common and were described as *"hypertrophy without valve disease"* [5]. Having made these anatomical observations, Bright put forward a novel hypothesis. *"The derangement of one organ is connected with the derangement of several others: yet we are not a liberty to assume, that the disease of the kidney has been the primary cause on which the disease of the rest depended. It may be, that some other organ has first suffered, and that the kidneys, together with the rest, have become involved. I confess I am inclined to believe that the kidney is the chief promoter of the other derangements"*. Bright's conception of a link between the anatomical alterations of the heart and kidneys via a pathophysiological mechanism (Bright would have said *"morbid derangement"*) as yet unknown, makes his publication the foundation stone of hypertension. Some articles on the history of medicine even claim that Richard Bright had suggested an elevation of blood pressure as the cause of left ventricular hypertrophy, but this may be an exaggeration [6]. In 1836, Bright did not yet have access to the experimental results which could have put him on the right track. As a second hypothesis for the causes of organ alterations, Bright imagined that skin disorders could be responsible. His reasoning was that a disease of the skin could account for all the anatomical findings by disrupting perspiration which would in turn explain the oedema and pleural effusions. With this interpretation, we were still a long way from the modern concept of "milieu intérieur" and blood pressure. Although Bright briefly alluded to the possibility of *"the chemical qualities of the blood"*, which were just beginning to be studied in the early days of medical chemistry, he had a tendency to minimise their importance. Finally, it should be noted that Bright's 100 cases were not 100 cases of hypertension but 100 cases of albuminuria [7].

There is, however, a general remark that Bright made about the renal diseases he observed which is worthy of mention because it introduces a concept which was taken up again and again and which was to remain true throughout the history of hypertension as well as many other chronic diseases discovered subsequently. *"The disease is often more advanced than we are led to believe when it first becomes the object of our attention: and I am most anxious, in the present communication, to impress upon*

5. Bright R. Tabular view of the morbid appearances in 100 cases connected with albuminous urine. With observations by Dr. Bright. *Guy's Hospital Reports* 1836, 1: 396.

6. The contribution of Richard Bright to the history of hypertension is often embellished by a retrospective analysis of historians. It is noteworthy that in the Dictionnaire encyclopédique des sciences médicales (Encyclopedic dictionary of medical sciences) edited by Dechambre at the end of the 19th century, and which is reputed to be one of the most accurate accounts of the current thinking of the time, the concept of blood pressure is not even mentioned in articles about Richard Bright or albuminuria, even though blood pressure manometers were already being used in laboratories at the time.

7. The youngest patient autopsied was 8 years old and the oldest was 73. Four were over the age of 60 and half the patients were aged between 30 and 40.

the members of our profession the insidious nature of this malady, that they may be led to watch its first approaches, with all the sollicitude which they would feel on discovering the first suspicious symptoms of phthisis or of epilepsy. There is great reason to suppose that the seeds of this disease are often sown at an early period; and that intervals of apparent health produce a false security in the patient, his friends, and his medical attendants, even where apprehension has been early excited" [8].

THE CONCEPT OF RENAL OBSTRUCTION AND CAPILLARY DISEASE: WHEN THEORY PRECEDES MEASUREMENT

Bright did not understand the anatomical finding of left ventricular hypertrophy and some 20 years later, Traube attempted to elucidate this problem. Unlike Bright, Traube had access to the latest results of the German physiologists who were at the leading edge in the mid-19th century, particularly Ludwig and his followers, working on blood pressure in dogs. Traube's contribution thus emanated from a physiological reasoning process rather than from an anatomico-clinical one. More clearly than Bright had done, he involved the notion of arterial hypertension in the description of a morbid process, that of renal failure in this case. In 1856, in a work on the relationship between cardiac and renal diseases, Traube elaborated a series of hypotheses based on a haemodynamic concept of the problem [9].

According to Traube, a *"renal obstruction"* induced a rise in blood pressure which in turn caused cardiac enlargement. *"The atrophy of the renal parenchyma [...] leads to a reduction in the quantity of liquid [...] removed from the circulatory system by urinary excretion. The inevitable result is that the blood pressure must rise"* [10].

Traube's reasoning (according to Vaquez) was the following :

1) In Bright's disease, there was a reduction in the size of the kidneys.
2) This led to a decrease in renal blood flow and therefore a reduction in total blood flow from the arteries to the veins.
3) There was also a reduction in urinary excretion.
4) The consequences of 2 and 3 (and especially 3) was an increase in mean arterial pressure.
5) The increase in pressure created a counter-force to the free flow of blood from the ventricle which therefore became dilated and then hypertrophied.

Traube explained his reasoning as follows: *"When a large quantity of blood is withdrawn from the vascular system of a dog, its blood pressure and its urinary excretion decrease about 30 minutes later. If defibrinated blood is then transfused back, the blood pressure increases as does the quantity of urine in the ureters. When the urinary volume declines, its mineral concentration increases"*.

8. Bright R. Cases and observations illustrative of renal disease accompanied with the secretion of albuminous urine. *Guy's Hospital Reports* 1836, 1: 338-379. This citation is also revelant to the "disappearance of symptoms" which will be discussed in chapter 7 — Yesterday's sufferers, today's patients.

9. Traube L. *Uber den Zuzammenhag von Herz und Nieren Krankheiten.* (Relationship between cardiac and renal diseases) 1871, Berlin.

10. This was a novel idea since at the time there was no way of measuring blood pressure in man. This is further proof that it is not measuring instruments that allow diseases to be conceived, but ideas.

In 1872, the English physicians William Gull and Gawen Sutton took a broader interest in the vascular system as a whole. Gull, like Bright, worked at Guy's Hospital and he was very familiar with this pathology on which he had already written several articles. But he was sceptical about the theory of the resistance of the renal arteries in left ventricular hypertrophy and arterial hypertension. According to Gull, the mechanism was a more general one since the arterioles *are more or less altered in the entire body* [11].

He expressed his scepticism with brio in the following terms: *"In this glass you see a much hypertrophied heart, and a very contracted kidney. This specimen is classical. It was, I believe, put up under Dr. Bright's own direction, and with a view of showing that the wasting of the kidney is the cause of the thickening of the heart. I cannot but look upon it with veneration, but not with conviction. I think, with all deference to so great an authority, that the systemic capillaries, and, had it been possible, the entire man, should have been included in this vase, together with the heart and the kidneys; and then we should have had, I believe, a truer view of the causation of the cardiac hypertrophy, and of the disease of the kidney"* [12].

Gull believed that it was the obliteration of the entire capillary system which accounted for the cardiac manifestations of Bright's disease. With this concept, Gull's thinking was along the lines of the German anatomopathologists who had described hypertensive nephroangiosclerosis [13].

Traube's concept was attractive and many clinicians began to speak of "Traube's heart" to describe the left ventricular hypertrophy observed in hypertension. But the pathophysiological mystery relating the heart and the kidneys could not simply be considered as a haemodynamic obstruction. After the anatomico-clinical era, then the haemodynamic era, endocrinology was about to enter the scene.

THE KIDNEY AND INTERNAL SECRETION: THE ERA OF ENDOCRINOLOGY

At the end of 19th century, when laboratory medicine and endocrinology were achieving their first successes, the idea of the *"internal secretion of the kidneys"* emerged. The *"milieu intérieur"* and the principle of *"internal secretion"* (Claude Bernard 1865) were amongst the modern concepts of medical science. In this context, Brown-Séquard published his *Experimental investigations into the physiology and pathology of the suprarenal glands* in 1856 and then went on to study the internal secretion of the testicle [14].

In 1889, in a presentation to the Society of Biology, he stated that: *"the excretory duct glands like the blood glands ("glandes sanguines") have an internal secretion"* and he quoted the kidney as an example. The basis of renal disease, he believed, was not solely defective filtration but also

11. Gull W., Sutton H.G., Chronic Bright's disease with contracted kidney. *Med Chir Trans* 1872; 55: 273-326.

12. Gull W. Clinical lecture on chronic Bright's disease with contracted kidney (arteriocapillary sclerosis). *Brit Med J* 1872; 2; 707-709.

13. Eald C.A. Ueber die Veränderungen Kleiner Gefässe bei Morbus Brighti und die darauf bezüglichen Therien. (Changes in small blood vessels in Bright's disease and theories thereof). *Virchows Arch Path Anat* 1877; 71: 453
Jores L. Ueber die Arteriosklerose der Kleinen Organarterien und ihre beziehungen zur Nephritis. (Arteriosclerosis of small vessels and its relationship to nephritis). *Virchows Arch Path Anat* 1904; 367.

14. After working in France and in the United States, Charles Brown-Séquard (1818-1894) replaced Claude Bernard at the College de France in 1878. A pioneer of endocrinology, his concept of internal secretion differed from that of Claude Bernard who invented the term. He foresaw the idea of

abnormalities of their internal secretion and of the renal nerves. In an article on *"The importance of the internal secretion of the kidneys revealed by the phenomenon of anuria and uraemia"* [15], Brown-Séquard expounded his theory. Although most of the details were not very accurate, this work set the stage for the discovery of renin by introducing the concept of renal secretion [16]. A new page in the history of medicine was about to be written: that of endocrinology. For the first 20 years of the 20th century, this new field met with success and failure and raised immense, and sometimes utopian therapeutic hope.

The discovery of the role of the endocrine glands was a major event. Against the background of therapeutic paucity, it had truly miraculous repercussions, exemplified by the treatment of hypothyroidism (Murray 1892) and above all of diabetes (discovery of insulin in 1922 by Banting, Best, Mac Leod and Collip). But the therapeutic use of hormones went far beyond simple hormone replacement therapy. Physicians sometimes used hormones excessively, incoherently, or even fraudulently. Hormone "deficiency" sprung up everywhere and there were even cases of tuberculosis being "treated" with ovarian extracts. Through shrewd advertising, hormone manufacturers encouraged these deficiencies, a source of quick and easy profits. Statistical analysis and control over the ethics of advertising were sorely lacking at the beginning of this century. So much so, in fact, that in 1922, the first reports of successful insulin therapy were met with suspicion by consciencious practitioners who were tired of reports of all sorts of miracles.

In the early 20th century, the prospect of endrocrine control raised immense hopes, some real, some totally imaginary. Blood pressure did not remain on the sidelines of this intense activity which was so profuse that it renders a historical analysis difficult.

THE DISCOVERY OF RENIN

Inspired by the work of Brown-Séquard, Tigerstedt, a Finnish physiologist, and Bergmann, a Swedish physician, performed a series of experiments in 1898 in an attempt to elucidate the relationship between the heart and the kidneys [17]. They injected fresh rabbit kidney homogenates, diluted in saline, into other animals. In their first experiment, the intravenous administration of the homogenates increased the blood pressure of a rabbit. Repeated injections into several animals consistently produced an increase in blood pressure. From their results, these authors deduced that their aqueous kidney extracts contained an active substance which they called "renin". They then went on to describe some of its physical and chemical properties. Pursuing their innovative work, they observed an elevation of blood pressure after injection of renal venous blood into rabbits who had undergone nephrectomy a day or two earlier. They concluded that *"a substance is formed in the kidneys which under normal conditions can pass into the bloodstream by a*

hormones in 1891, although the word itself appeared only in 1905.

15. *Archives de physiologie.* 1893, p. 778.

16. This approach was to have considerable repercussions in the area of hypertension. Using the method, Oliver and Schäfer discovered the strong hypertensive action of adrenal gland extracts in 1894. Tigerstedt and Bergmann, the discoverers of renin, also quote Brown-Séquard. The conclusion to Brown-Séquard's article quoted by Tigerstedt and Bergmann (*Archives de physiologie* 1893. p. 778) was the following:
1. *"If one confronts the observations of long-standing anuria, without morbid manifestations, and the disappearance of the symptoms due to nephrectomy, under the influence of injections of renal extract, it is clear that the kidney is endowed with an extremely important capacity for internal secretion.*
2. *A comparative study of anuria and uraemia [...] makes it highly probable that the phenomenon of uraemia is due essentially to the absence of renal internal secretion and not, as is sometimes believed, to the alteration of urinary secretion and the ensuing accumulation of certain toxic substances in the blood".*

17. Tigerstedt R., Bergmann P.G. Niere und Kreislauf (The kidney and the circulation) *Scand Arch Physiol* 1898; 8: 223-271.

process of internal secretion and exert a hypertensive effect" [18]. At the end of 19th century, the existence of renin was definitively acknowledged.

Author of three lectures published in The Lancet in May 1906, Batty Shaw referred to the work of Tigerstedt in a review of the literature on the relationships between the kidney, hypertension and cardiovascular disease [19]. At that time, it was established that only extracts of the adrenal gland, the kidney, and the posterial lobe of the pituitary gland induced an increase in blood pressure. While there was general agreement that the adrenal gland exerted its effect via the secretion of adrenaline into the blood, opinions differed about renin because it had not been possible to reproduce Tigerstedt's observations. On the basis of personal experience, Batty Shaw remarked that a substance extracted from the renal cortex was capable of raising blood pressure and provided an explanation for the commonly observed hypertrophy of the tunica media of the arteries and of the heart.

From this stage on, it appeared likely that the kidney, in addition to the established role of the adrenal glands, could be responsible for hypertension. For over 30 years, many investigators attempted to raise the blood pressure of laboratory animals by different types of manipulations of the kidney. These included the injection of nephrotoxic products, irradiation of the kidneys, clamping of renal vessels, and partial nephrectomies, with or without ligation of the branches of the renal artery. They met with variable degrees of success in their venture to prove the responsibility of the kidney in hypertension [20].

GOLDBLATT INVENTS A FORM OF EXPERIMENTAL HYPERTENSION... HIS REPORT IS REJECTED BY THE AMERICAN HEART JOURNAL

It was in Germany that the first experimental protocols were designed to test the theory of the role of the kidney in hypertension. Paul Grawitz and Oscar Israel embarked on this venture by creating a complete obstruction of a renal artery in rabbits for periods ranging from half an hour to two hours. The animals were then observed for several days or weeks before being autopsied. The kidneys and heart were weighed and showed cardiac enlargement in aged animals. Unfortunately, the manometric measurements (performed invasively in the carotid artery) did not show a rise in blood pressure and so, Grawitz and Israel fell just wide of the mark of experimental hypertension. Their idea of blocking the renal circulation would have been a good one however had they been more insistent and used a species other than the rabbit. Ludwig Lewinski, first assistant at the Polyclinic in Berlin, was more fortunate. He constricted the two renal arteries of a dog without totally interrupting renal blood flow and was thus able to verify the relationship between renal disease and cardiac enlargement. Lewinski however was unable

18. *" We wish only to emphasise that the substance we have obtained from the kidneys could play an important role in the cardiac enlargement observed in certain renal diseases. We cannot rule out the possibility that this substance might, under certain circumstances, be produced in excess and excreted more slowly than normally and thereby increase vessel resistance above its normal value. The consequence would be cardiac enlargement. This being said, we wish to emphasise that we are not proposing a new hypothesis to explain the relationship between cardiac enlargement and renal disease. [...] We simply wish to draw attention to the possible significance of a renal substance which increases blood pressure. We cannot be sure whether renin acts on the vascular nerve centers of the spinal cord. However, under certain circumstances, there is an extremely powerful effect of renin on the peripheral nerve centres of blood vessels. Finally, renin has no direct effect on blood vessels"*.

19. *"A substance extracted from the renal cortex and capable of increasing blood pressure was discovered by Tigerstedt and Bergmann [...]. Their clinical and experimental findings support the hypothesis that permanent hypertension could be due to the presence in the circulation of a substance of renal origin [...]. The action of the renal substance, by increasing blood pressure, provides an explanation for the commonly observed hypertrophy of the tunica media of the arteries and of the heart"*. Batty Shaw H. Auto-intoxication: its relation to certain disturbances of blood pressure. *Lancet* 1906, pp. 1295-1306: 1375-1380; and 1455-1462.

20. For more information, see David B. Gordon. Some early investigations of experimental hypertension. An historical review. *Texas Rep Biol Med* 1970; 28: 3.

to confirm Traube's intuition that there would be a hypertensive mechanism, probably on account of some technical problem which led him to omit manometric measurements from his experiments. Many other authors then set about the task of trying to achieve experimental hypertension. These included Katzenstein, Wood, Dominguez, Hartman, Pedersen, Janeway and Cash. They clamped, incised, irradiated, ligated and injected nephrotoxic substances into the renal arteries. In 1925, the German investigator, Fahr, who was the first to describe malignant hypertension, alluded to the problem of "renal ischaemia".

It was not until the work of Harry Goldblatt that a reliable experimental model was finally achieved. Having noticed that at autopsy many hypertensive patients exhibited abnormalities of the intrarenal arteries, Goldblatt decided to explore once again the now classical hypothesis of the renal origin of hypertension. Unable to manipulate the intrarenal arteries directly, Goldblatt decided in 1934 to perform a bilateral stenosis of the renal arteries. His experimental protocol proved to be more effective than that of his predecessors. To control the degree of stenosis, he developed a ingenious device capable of achieving variable degrees of constriction of the renal arteries and he observed the level of the systolic blood pressure measured in the carotid artery. The renal function of the dogs was assessed by measuring the clearance of urea and the excretion of phenolsulfonphthalein. Through his very careful experimental technique, Goldblatt achieved the first reliable and reproducible experimental model. He thus discovered that hypertension created by stenosis of the renal arteries could be observed even without changes in renal function or renal necrosis.Control experiments showed that constricting the splenic artery, the femoral artery or the carotid artery did not induce an elevation of blood pressure. Goldblatt did not cite Tigerstedt and Bergmann in his first publication [21].

He proposed 3 pathophysiological hypotheses:
(1) A nerve impulse originating in the nerves of the ischaemic kidneys could be propagated to the sympathetic ganglia or to a vasomotor center and could induce generalised vasoconstriction and a rise in blood pressure.
(2) This nerve impulse could stimulate an internal secretion, which, by a central or peripheral action, could induce generalised vasoconstriction and a rise in blood pressure.
(3) There could be accumulation or formation of a substance, or an imbalance between substances in the blood, which could exert a hormone-like hypertensive effect.

More than 30 years after the work of Tigerstedt and Bergmann, it did not take Goldblatt very long to show that the third hypothesis was the right one and today his name is definitively connected with the history of renovascular hypertension [22].

21. Goldblatt H., Lynch J., Hanzal R.F., Summerville W.W. Studies on experimental hypertension. 1. The production of persistent elevation of systolic blood pressure by means of renal ischemia. *J Exp Med* 1934; 59: 347-379.

22. Goldblatt H. Hypertension due to renal ischemia. *Bull N.Y. Acad Med* 1964; 40: 745-758.
(The Third Ferdinand C. Valentine Memorial Lecture, delivered before the Section on Urology of the New York Academy of Medicine, March 21, 1964).

The importance of this discovery, however, was not immediately obvious because at the time cardiologists were not particularly well disposed to the jargon of the physiologists. And so it happened that the *American Heart Journal* rejected Goldbatt's paper which he then sent to the *Journal of Experimental Medicine*.

FROM "HYPERTENSIN" TO THE RENIN-ANGIOTENSIN SYSTEM: THE ERA OF BIOLOGY

Once a reliable animal model of renovascular hypertension had been achieved, research into a hypertensive renal factor entered the modern era. Progress in the understanding of the renin-angiotensin system derived from a multi-disciplinary collaboration between physiologists, biochemists, anatomists, clinicians and molecular biologists. It took only a few decades for the renin-angiotensin system to be dissected in detail.

Shortly after Goldblatt's publication, several groups showed that renin was not the actual vasopressive hormone. It exerted its effect by releasing a vasopressive peptide from a plasma precursor. The groups of Braun-Menendez in Argentina and Page in Cleveland referred to this peptide respectively as hypertensin and angiotonin before finally agreeing on the name angiotensin [23].

The isolation and composition of angiotensin was achieved simultaneously on both sides of the Atlantic by Skeggs et al. in the U.S. and by Peart and his colleagues in England [24]. Skeggs et al. made a further important contribution when they demonstrated the action of the converting enzyme which split off the histidyl-leucine dipeptide from angiotensin I to form angiotensin II, an octapeptide which is much more biologically active. Angiotensin II was synthesised by Schwyzer et al. in 1956. In 1957, Elliot and Peart on the one hand, and Skeggs and his coworkers on the other, determined the amino acid sequences of equine and bovine angiotensins. Once desoxycorticosterone had been synthesised, it was quickly shown that this steroid, which affected sodium and potassium metabolism, could induce hypertension in both animals and man. An important point was that this hypertension was sodium-dependent, unlike the hypertension induced by the glucocorticoids. The discovery of aldosterone by Simpson in 1953 and the development of an assay for its urinary determination paved the way for a more detailed study of its metabolism [25].

In the early 1950s, Luetscher and Axelrad performed a series of experiments to investigate the mechanism by which sodium deprivation was associated with a decrease in its urinary excretion [26]. They observed an inverse relationship between aldosterone and the urinary excretion

23. Muñoz J.M., Braun-Menéndez E., Fasciolo J.C., Leloir L.F. Hypertensin: the substance causing renal hypertension. *Nature* 1939; 144: 980.
Page I.H. Helmer O.M. A crystalline pressor substance (angiotonin) resulting from the action between renin and renin-activator. *J Exp Med* 1940; 71: 29-282.
Braun-Menéndez E. and Page I.H. Suggested revision of nomenclature — angiotensin. *Science* N.Y. 1958, 127: 242

24. Skeggs L.T., Marsh W.H. Kahn J.R., Shumway N.P. The existence of two forms of hypertensin. *J Exp Med* 1954; 99: 275-282.
Peart W.S. et al. A new method of large-scale preparation of hypertensin with a note on its assay. *Biochem J* 1954; 59:300

25. Simpson S.A., Tait J.F. Wettstein A., Neher R., Von Heuw J. and Reichstein T. Isolieurung eines neuen kristallisierten Hormons aus Nebennieren mit besonders hoher Wirksamkeit auf den Mineralstoff-Wechsel. (Isolation of a new crystalline adrenal hormone with strong activity on mineral exchange) *Experientia* (Bale) 1953; 9:333.

26. Luetscher J.A., Axelrad B.J. Increased aldosterone output during sodium deprivation in normal men. *Proc Soc Exp Biol Med* 1954; 87: 650-653.

of sodium. In 1954, in a study of two healthy volunteers they further showed that:

(1) sodium retention could not be explained by a reduction in glomerular filtration, and especially that

(2) the secretion of aldosterone was independent of the secretion of ACTH. It now remained to discover the factor which stimulated the production of aldosterone.

After being the object of intense study in pathological situations (hypertensive disease) renin and angiotensin began to attract the attention of physiologists after Franz Gross showed that the renin-angiotensin system also plays a role in the normal individual. In 1954, Sulser and Gross showed that the vasopressive effects of administering renin to rats were comparable regardless of whether hypertension was induced by the administration of salt and desoxycorticosterone or nephrectomy. They put forward the hypothesis that a common mechanism — the disappearance of renin — accounted for this result. They confirmed this hypothesis by showing that the kidneys of rats treated with salt and desoxycorticosterone failed to secrete renin-like vasopressive substances. Gross then proposed, in 1958, a mechanism linking the secretions of renin and aldosterone [27].

In 1960 and 1961, Davis, Genest and Laragh showed that the administration of angiotensin II increased the secretion of aldosterone in both dogs and man. This confirmed Gross's hypothesis. Little by little, the hormonal regulation of blood pressure was revealing some of its secrets [28].

As physiology moved forward, histology also made its contribution. Back in 1925, Ruyter had described juxtaglomerular cells as cells derived from muscle cells [29]. Twenty years later, Goormaghtigh demonstrated the endocrine nature of the cells and finally Hartroft and Hartroft showed that there was a good correlation between the renin content of the kidney and the degree of granulation of the juxtaglomerular cells [30]. But it was only in 1961 that renin was shown to be present directly in the granules of juxtaglomerular cells by means of a fluorescent-antibody technique [31].

The answer to the burning question of the aetiology of hypertension was coming closer thanks to the improved understanding of the renin-angiotensin-aldosterone system. Thus the description by Conn in 1955 of a form of arterial hypertension with hypokalaemia and aldosteronism (which today bears his name) and the discovery of renin-secreting tumours in 1967 were made in a context of significantly improved understanding of the endocrine system.

27. Gross F. Renin und Hypertensin, physiologishe oder pathologische Wirkstoffe? (Renin and hypertensin. Physiologic or pathologic substances?) *Klin Wochenschr* 1958; 36: 693-706.

28. Laragh J.H., Angers M., Kelly W.G., Lieberman S. Hypotensive agents and pressor substances. The effect of epinephrine, norepinephrine, angiotensin II and others on the secretory rate of aldosterone in man. *JAMA* 1960; 174: 243-240.
Davis J.O. Mechanisms regulating the secretion and metabolism of aldosterone in experimental secondary hyperaldosteronism. *Recent Prog Horm Res* 1961; 17: 293-352.
Genest J., Nowaczynski W., Koiw E., Sandor T., Biron P. Adrenocortical function in essential hypertension. in: *Essential Hypertension*, Bock K.D. and Cottier P.T. 1960 Springer-Verlag, Berlin. pp. 126-146.

29. Ruyter J.H.C. Uber einen merkwurdigen abschnitt der vasa afferentia in der mauseniere. (On an unusual afferent vessel structure in murine kidney) *Z Zellforsh Mikrosk Anat* 1925; 2: 242-248.

30. Goormaghtigh N. La fonction endocrine des artérioles rénales. Son rôle dans la pathogénie de l'hypertension artérielle (The endocrine function of renal arterioles. Its role in the pathogenesis of arterial hypertension). *Rev Belge Sci Méd* 1944-1945. 16: 65-83.
Hartroft P.M., Hartroft W.S. Studies on renal juxtaglomerular cells, I. Variations produced by sodium chloride and desoxycorticosterone acetate. *J Exp Med* 1953; 97: 415-427.
Hartroft P.M. Hartroft W.S. Studies on renal juxtaglomerular cells, II. Correlation of the degree of granulation of juxtaglomerular cells with width of the zona glomerulosa of the adrenal cortex. *J Exp Med* 1955; 12: 205-212.

31. Edelman R., Hartroft P.M. Localization of renin in juxtaglomerular cells of rabbit and dog through use of the fluorescent-antibody technique. *Circ Res* 1961; 9: 1069-1077.

1960-1970: THERAPY WITHIN SIGHT

By the mid-1960s, considerable progress had been made. The main elements of the physiology of the renin-angiotensin-aldosterone system had been elucidated and so called secondary forms of hypertension had been described at the two extremities of the system, i.e. by excessive or inappropriate secretion of renin (malignant hypertension, renovascular hypertension) and by excessive aldosterone secretion (Conn's syndrome). Today, researchers are turning their attention to so-called essential hypertension. Some believe that there is clinical and experimental evidence to suggest the possible involvement of renin. Whether this is true or not, only the future will tell.

Pheochromocytoma and the concept of
surgically curable hypertension

"In the final analysis, despite our reservations on the interpretation of this particularly puzzling and heretofore unique case, or so we believe, we would tend to consider all the symptoms of this disease, that is the paroxysmal hypertension, the solar and vasocontrictive crises, the tachycardia and the sympatheticotonic signs as the expression of a state of acute adrenalism caused by the development of a tumour with characteristics of the adrenal medulla".

M. Labbé, 1922 [1]

Pheochromocytoma was the first known cause of curable hypertension. Fränkel described the symptoms and the tumour of the adrenal gland in 1886 [2]. A quarter of a century later, progress in technical and biological knowledge was such that Labbé et al. were able to give a complete description of the disease and a correct interpretation of its pathophysiology [1]. The earliest resection of a pheochromocytoma dates back to 1927 [3], in a patient whose tumour was not diagnosed preoperatively. The first operation based on a preoperative diagnosis with the stated aim of normalising blood pressure was performed 1929 [4]. By comparison, renovascular hypertension was induced in dogs in 1934 [5] and demonstrated in man in 1937 [6]. Conn described primary aldosteronism only in 1955 [7].

NEPHRITIS WITH A SUPRARENAL TUMOUR

Retrospectively, it appears that credit for the first description of pheochromocytoma should go to Fränkel. In 1886, that is at a time when clinicians were unaware of the concept of hypertension and when blood pressure was not measured at the bedside, this author reported the case of an 18-year-old girl hospitalised for declining visual acuity and weight loss [2]. She complained of headaches, palpitations and sweating with a markedly paroxysmal course. At times, she was pale and prostrate while at other times, she was relaxed *"and sung with the other patients"*. Clinical examination revealed tachycardia and paleness. The urine contained abundant amounts of protein and her fundus showed abnormalities (consistent with what would be considered today as stage IV hypertensive

1. Labbé M., Tinel J., Doumer A. Crises solaires et hypertension paroxystique en rapport avec une tumeur surrénale (Solar crises and paroxysmal hypertension related to an adrenal tumour). *Bull Soc Med Hôp* 1922; 46: 982- 990.

2. Fränkel F. Ein fall von doppelseitigem, völlig latent verlaufenen nebennierentumor und gleichzeitiger nephritis mit veränderungen am circulationsapparat und retinitis. (A case of a bilateral suprarenal tumour with a latent course, accompanied by nephritis, circulatory changes and retinitis). *Virchow Arch Path Anat* 1886; 103: 244-263.

3. Mayo C. Paroxysmal hypertension with tumor of retroperitoneal nerve. *JAMA* 1927; 139: 1047- 1050.

4. Pincoffs M.C. A case of paroxysmal hypertension associated with a suprarenal tumor. *Trans Assoc Am Phys* 1929; 44: 295-299.

5. Goldblatt H., Lynch J., Hanzal R.F. Studies on experimental hypertension I: The production of persistent elevation of systolic blood pressure by means of renal ischemia. *J Exp Med* 1934; 59: 347-379.

6. Butler A.M. Chronic pyelonephritis and arterial hypertension. *J Clin Invest* 1937; 16: 889-897.

7. Conn J.W. Primary aldosteronism, a new clinical sydnrome. *J Lab Clin Med* 1955; 43:6-17.

retinopathy). She died in spite of the administration of ether, tartrate, digitalis, pilocarpine and even medicinal wine (alcohol was still considered as medicine). The autopsy showed an enlarged heart, macroscopically normal kidneys and a tumour of both suprarenal glands 8 cm in diameter on the left and 1 cm on the right. The large tumour was mobile, non-homogenous, haemorrhagic and greyish-brown in colour. Because of its highly vascular nature, it was diagnosed as an angiosarcoma.

A CASE OF PAROXYSMAL HYPERTENSION WITH A SUPRARENAL TUMOUR: "SOLAR CRISES" SUGGESTING " A STATE OF HYPERADRENALISM"

The first publication which presented an explicit description and commentary of pheochromocytoma was that of Labbé et al. in 1922 [1]. More than thirty years had passed since the observation of Fränkel and the intellectual context had changed radically because the concept of hypertension was now well established. Labbé reported the case of a 28-year-old woman hospitalised for paroxysmal attacks of epigastric constriction with headaches, sweating, palpitations and vomiting during which Pachon's sphygmomanometer recorded systolic pressures as high as 280 mmHg. Her systolic blood pressure varied from 125 to 280 mmHg, was always elevated during the attacks and sometimes even during the intervening periods. Laboratory tests showed the presence of proteinuria, glycosuria and intermittent hyperazotaemia. Because of the sympatheticotonic appearance of the crises, an adrenaline test was performed with the idea of reproducing the spontaneous symptoms to confirm the responsibility of this vasopressive amine. Within a few minutes, the injection of 1 mg of adrenaline induced a mild elevation of blood pressure from 155 to 165 mmHg without acceleration of the pulse and without horripilation. It also induced fairly persistent glycosuria.[8] The course was complicated by three episodes of acute pulmonary oedema and death ensued. Autopsy revealed a tumour of the left suprarenal gland about 6 cm in diameter arising from the "*suprarenal medullary substance, [...] an authentic paraganglioma*".

On the basis of recently acquired knowledge in both endocrinology and cardiovascular medicine, Labbé and his coworkers proposed a pathophysiological mechanism for their observation. They recognised that the highly vascular tumour with its syncytial appearance was of medullary origin. Since 1895, it had been known that the adrenal medulla secreted amines which, when injected into animals, increased blood pressure [9]. This was the case in particular of adrenaline, synthesised by Stolz in 1904 [10]. Labbé explained that he was "*unable to show a positive Vulpian test, characteristic of adrenaline*" but he felt that the clinical and pathological picture was sufficiently explicit.

8. This inconstant effect is attributed today to the down-regulation of alpha receptors in pheochromocytoma. Snavely M.D., Mahan L.C., O'Connor D.T., Insel P.A. Selective down-regulation of adrenergic receptor subtypes in tissues from rats with pheochromocytoma. *Endocrinology* 1983; 113: 354-361.

9. Oliver G., Schäfer E.A. Physiological effects of extracts of the suprarenal capsules. *J. Physiol* (London) 1895; 18: 230.

10. Stolz GF. Ueber adrenalin und alkylaminoacetobenzcatechin. (Adrenaline and alkyl-amino-acetobenzo-catecholamine) *Ber Deutsch Chem Ges* 1904; 37: 41-49.

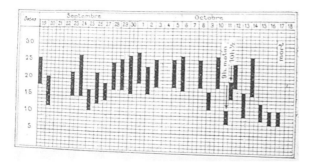

1

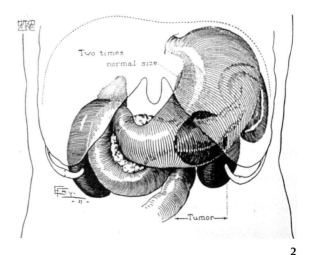

2

Pheochromocytoma: a surgically curable cause of hypertension

In 1922, Labbé, Tinel and Doumer published an observation of *"paroxysmal arterial hypertension with solar crises related to a suprarenal tumour"* in the Bulletin de la Société Médicale des Hôpitaux de Paris. The blood pressure variations were well documented (figure1) and were reminiscent of a case previously published by Vaquez. The patient was 28 years of age and died of cardiorespiratory failure after 7 months of observation. In 1927, the American surgeon Charles Mayo reported in the JAMA the case of a 30-year-old female music teacher who presented with paroxysmal episodes of hypertension. The systolic blood pressure often exceeded 300 mmHg with a diastolic exceeding 180 mmHg and maximum pressures of 320 mmHg. Because of the uncertainty as to diagnosis, she was admitted to hospital for observation for several weeks. The attacks, which had begun a year previously, continued with nausea, vomiting, dyspnea, exhaustion and visual disturbances. Prostration and abdominal pain ensued but the patient never lost consciousness. A number of different drugs were tried (digitalis, quinidine, amyl nitrite, bromide, choral, phenobarbital, belladona, potassium iodide, morphine, antityphoid vaccination, histamine) but all proved to be ineffective. Because of the belief that the symptoms were is some way *"mediated through the sympathetic nervous system"*, the decision was made to operate with the intention of severing the splanchnic nerves. After a large medial incision, the surgeon was surprised to discover a retroperitoneal mass 6 by 4 cm which had not been detected on clinical examination (figure 2). The diagnosis of *"malignant retroperitoneal blastoma"* was made. Importantly, following resection of the tumour, the blood pressure fell to around 120 mmHg and the patient regained weight. In his publication, Mayo did not really provide a pathophysiological interpretation but in his bibliography he cited the previous observations of Labbé and Vaquez. Two years after Mayo's report, Pincoffs confronted with a similar case, made a preoperative diagnosis of the possible role of an adrenaline-secreting tumour.

He referred to the tumour as a "*paraganglioma*" and did not use the term pheochromocytoma [11]. Labbé concluded: "*We would be inclined to consider that all the symptoms of this disease, paroxysmal hypertension, solar and vasoconstrictive crises, tachycardia and a state of sympathe-ticotonia, as the expression of a state of acute hyperadrenalinaemia resulting from the development of a tumour exhibiting the characteristics of the medullary substance of the adrenal gland*". Thus, the concept of a tumour able to induce hypertension arose. Two weeks after Labbé's communication, Aubertin, in a presentation to the Hospital Medical Society on June 23rd, 1922, commented that "*The patient described by Doctors Labbé, Tinel and Doumer might be considered as the first case of a new syndrome of paroxysmal hypertension of adrenal origin*". And yet, Vaquez and Aubertin in 1907 as well as Laignel-Lavastine and Aubertin himself in 1908 had diagnosed possible suprarenal tumours responsible for paroxysmal hypertension. Their contributions should not be forgotten [12].

REMOVAL OF THE TUMOUR SUPRESSES HYPERTENSION

It took five years to progress from observation to action. In 1927, Mayo reported paroxysmal hypertension in a young woman whose systolic blood pressure often exceeded 300mmHg with a diastolic blood pressure exceeding 180mmHg and vasomotor disturbances [3]. With the availability of new possibilities for the surgical treatment of malignant hypertension, Mayo decided to operate with the idea that splanchnic neurectomy could improve the blood pressure variability. To his surprise, he found a 6 x 4 cm mass above the left kidney which had not been noted on clinical examination. The tumour was a greyish colour on resection and turned yellowish-orange after fixation with formaldehyde giving it the appearance of a corticoadrenal adenoma, but the characteristic differentiated cells with their gland-like arrangement was missing. Mayo's diagnosis was "*a retroperitoneal malignant blastoma*". He decided against sympathectomy and proceeded to resect the tumour. Post-operatively, he noted a return to normal of the blood pressure and the patient put on 30 pounds. His publication makes no mention of pathophysiology.

The credit for suspecting, then confirming an adrenaline-secreting tumour in a similar case, must go to Pincoffs, who noted that the "*abrupt rise in blood pressure, the evident peripheral vasoconstriction, the patient's nervous tremors, the violent activity of the heart and the glycosuria all indicated the action of adrenaline*" [4]. He first operated on the patient's left adrenal gland with no result but then on the right, he found what he was looking for: an adrenal tumour which stained positively for adrenaline. He thus confirmed the causal relationship between the adrenal medullary tumour, the release of adrenaline and hypertension with paroxysmal vasomotor disturbances. He then went

11. The term "*paraganglioma*" is usually used to refer to extra-adrenal pheochromocytomas. The term pheochromocytoma, proposed in 1912 by Pick corresponds to tumours of the adrenal medulla which blacken on contact with fixatives containing bichromate. Pick L. Das ganglioma embryonale sympathicum (sympathoma embryonale). *Berl Klin Wochenschr* 1912; 49: 16-22.

12. Vaquez and Aubertin. Coeur de Traube et hyperplasie médullaire des surrénales. (Traube's heart and medullary hyperplasia of the suprarenal glands) *Session reports of the Society of Biology*. May 25th 1907. pp. 967-969.
Laignel-Lavastine and Aubertin. Médullome surrénal (suprarenal medulloma). *Arch de méd expérimentale et d'anat pathol*, November 1908.

on to confirm that blood pressure returned permanently to normal after the operation. Previously suspected, this time the causal relationship between a tumour and hypertension was firmly established.

SLOW PROGRESS IN DIAGNOSTIC TECHNIQUES

By the end of the 1920s, the anatomico-clinical picture of paroxysmal hypertension of adrenal origin was well defined and its pathophysiological mechanism was clear: the rise in blood pressure and the vasomotor disturbances were the expression of an intermittent secretion of adrenal medullary catecholamines. This syndrome offered the prospect of cure by surgery, which was indicated on two counts: to remove the tumour but also to eradicate the symptoms, lower blood pressure and restore general health [3, 4]. But at the time, there were still formidable obstacles to the adoption of these concepts into everyday medical practice, notably because of the rareness of this disorder [13].

For many years, the diagnosis of a "acute hyperadrenalism" remained a clinical one. The patients of Labbé, Mayo and Pincoffs all had severe hypertension and a very striking clinical picture. It is probable that many less typical cases went undiagnosed. Furthermore, in view of the high operative risk at the time, it took great courage both on the part of the surgeon and the patient to follow the example of Mayo and Pincoffs. What were sorely lacking were tests to confirm the diagnosis preoperatively. These tests would only become available after the Second World War.

The first available test was pharmacological. We have already seen that the adrenaline test attempted by Labbé in 1922, then by Pincoffs in 1929, had not successfully reproduced the spontaneous paroxysmal bouts. Attention was then turned to empirical provocation tests which released catecholamines from the tumour or stored in extra-tumoral reuptake sites. This was the histamine test described in 1945 [14], followed through to the 1970s by tests using other substances including benzodioxane, tetraethyl-ammonium, tyramine, glucagon, propranolol, sulpiride, etc. The principle of these tests was to induce a bout of hypertension. The result was assessed on the basis of a blood pressure gradient (a histamine test was considered positive if the blood pressure rose by at least 60/40 mmHg). These tests were associated with a certain degree of morbidity or even mortality, and many considered them too dangerous to be used.

The measurement of urinary catecholamines and their metabolites, vanyllmandelic acid and metanephrines, became available in 1950 [15]. In 1970, a reproducible technique for measuring plasma catecholamines was described [16]. Surprisingly, the provocation test continued to be used long after the development of tests for quantifying the release of

13. Fifty years after Mayo's first operation, his successors observed 54 pheochromocytomas out of a total 40,078 autopsies performed at the Mayo clinic i.e. a prevalence of 0.13%. In 41 of these 54 subjects (76%) the diagnosis had not been made prior to death.
Sutton M.G., Sheps S.G., Lie J.T. Prevalence of clinically unsuspected pheochromocytoma. Review of a 50-year autopsy series. *Mayo Clin Proc* 1981; 56: 354-360.

14. Roth G.M., Kvale W.F. A tentative test for pheochromocytoma. *Am J Med Sci* 1945; 210: 653-700.

15. Engel A., von Euler U.S. Diagnostic value of increased urinary output of adrenaline and noradrenaline in pheochromocytoma. *Lancet* 1950; II: 387.

16. Engelman K., Portnoy B., Sjoerdsma A. Plasma catecholamine concentrations in patients with hypertension. *Circ Res* 1970; 26-27 (suppl. I): I-141-145.

endogenous catecholamines. It is true that these tests can be negative when the patient is not in a crisis, so that normal levels of catecholamines do not rule out the diagnosis of pheochromocytoma unless the patient's blood pressure is elevated: this is Engelman's rule [17]. This may appear to justify provocation tests in patients with an intermittently secreting pheochromocytoma, but in fact these tests also give false negative results in patients whose blood pressure and catecholamine levels are normal on the day of the test [18]. History does not tell us how many of these indirect tests led to complications or useless surgical interventions...

Another major difficulty was actually locating the tumour [19]. We know today that 90% of pheochromocytomas are situated in the adrenal glands and that they occur twice as frequently on the right than on the left for reasons which remain mysterious. Pincoffs' patient had a right adrenal pheochromocytoma but she first underwent a left sub-costal incision, no doubt because in the cases of Labbé and Mayo, the tumour was on the left! This stroke of bad luck did not prevent her from being cured two weeks later by the resection of the right adrenal gland. Apart from the 9% of palpable pheochromocytomas [12], until the 1950s the only methods of diagnosis were plain abdominal films and then tomography combined with urography or a retropneumoperitoneum, not very reliable techniques and not without danger. As recently as 1977, Engelman wrote that accurate preoperative localisation of a pheochromocytoma was really only a problem for the inexperienced surgeon. Engelman's attitude was that definite biochemical evidence was sufficient to prompt the surgeon to perform a medial laparotomy in the course of which he could identify the tumour, if not by inspection of the retroperitoneum, then by its palpation because contact with the tumour triggered a rise in blood pressure [17].

In the years that followed, tomodensitometry, scintigraphy and magnetic resonance imaging became available. These methods made it possible to localise the tumour preoperatively with an accuracy approaching 100% and, like the progress in anaesthesia, contributed to the improved safety of patients and peace of mind of the surgeon...

AN ERA OF NEW UNCERTAINTY ?

In experienced hands, with modern biochemical and imaging support, today's patients can expect almost perfect diagnostic accuracy and operative safety. The improved prognosis for patients undergoing surgery for pheochromocytoma has created new uncertainty concerning the long-term outcome. There is some evidence to suggest that the ten-year recurrence rate of benign or malignant tumours could be as high as 25%. Looked at in this light, can we still consider the discovery of pheochromocytoma as a fortunate event for the hypertensive patient and

17. Engelman K. Pheochromo-cytoma. *Clin Endocrinol Metab* 1977; 6: 769-797.

18. Sheps S.G., Maher F.T. Histamine and glucagon tests in the diagnosis of pheochromocytoma. *JAMA* 1968. 205: 895-899.

19. This was also a problem with primary hyperaldosteronism.

is this really a curable cause of hypertension? Progress in our understanding of tumorigenesis and the mechanisms of metastatic spread might provide prognostic and even preventive solutions to these problems. The history of pheochromocytoma is far from over.

The chronology of discoveries in pheochromocytoma research

1886   Fränkel describes the association of an adrenal tumour with a clinical picture of nephritis and retinitis [1].

1895   Oliver and Schäfer demonstrate that extracts from the adrenal medulla induce elevation of blood pressure in animals [9].

1904   Stolz synthesises adrenaline [10].

1912   Pick uses the term "*pheochromocytoma*" to designate tumours of the adrenal medulla which blacken with fixatives containing bichromate [11].

1922   Labbé et al. describe and explain paroxysmal hypertension in a patient with a tumour of the adrenal medulla [2].

1927   Mayo successfully resects a "*tumour of a retroperitoneal nerve*" [3].

1929   Pincoffs operates on a preoperatively suspected pheochromocytoma and confirms the normalisation of blood pressure post-operatively [4].

1950   Engel and von Euler measure urinary catecholamines [15].

Conn and aldosteronism

"You see, gentlemen, there is quite a difference between the scientist who observes and the artist who creates".

Armand Trousseau
Hôtel-Dieu hospital
Paris. 1861

In April 1954, a 34-year-old woman suffering from severe hypertension, was referred to the endocrinologist Jerome Conn at Ann Arbor in Michigan. He undertook a series of sophisticated biological investigations which enabled him to show that there was marked sodium retention with concomitant urinary potassium loss [1]. Having observed high levels of aldosterone in the urine, Conn suggested an unprecedented hypothesis: *"In 1954, after 8 months of close and continual observation of a single patient, I came to a new conclusion: this hypertensive patient is suffering from a hitherto unknown disease due to the excessive production of a recently discovered hormone, aldosterone"*. In his own words, Conn *"temporarily"* referred to this *"unknown disease"* as *"primary aldosteronism"*.

It thus took 8 months of observation and investigation for Conn to reach this conclusion which remains a model of scientific reasoning based on a single clinical case. Conn's discovery took the role of the adrenal cortex from one of theoretical confusion to that of clinical reality in which a hypersecreting adenoma was responsible for a clinical syndrome, dominated by symptomatic hypertension.

The correctness of Conn's reasoning was confirmed by the disappearance of clinical symptoms following surgical resection of the endocrine tumour, indisputable proof of causality. By his clinical deduction, Conn made a major contribution to our knowledge of the regulatory mechanisms of blood pressure, well before the development of sophisticated biochemical techniques for studying steroids. But let us make no mistake, Conn's brilliant discovery was not due to the good fortune of having observed an exemplary patient [2]. It was above all the reward of an alert and well-prepared mind: *"My intense interest in the phenomenon to be described stems from work carried out in my laboratory from 1943 to 1948"* stated Conn in his original description. The regulation of salt and corticosteroids was indeed an area with which he was very familiar. Five years previously

1. Conn J.W. Primary aldosteronism, a new clinical syndrome. *J Lab Clin Med* 1955; 4: 661-664.

2. Primary aldosteronism is relatively rare, estimated today to affect 1% of a non-selected hypertensive population. There is reason to believe that previously it was even lower, or possibly "concealed" by the fact that secondary hyperaldosteronism was relatively common (heart failure, cirrhosis, etc.).

he had written: *"Changes in the concentration of sodium and chloride of thermal sweat, collected under standard conditions, parallels changes in the activity of the adrenal cortex with respect to its elaboration of steroids which act like desoxycorticosterone. The ability to observe changes in activity of salt-active corticoids is of potential value in investigative medicine, in elucidating the possible role of the salt-active corticoids in a wide variety of clinical conditions, nephrosis, congestive heart failure, essential hypertension, premenstrual edema"* [3]. During this period it was shown that the urine of patients with renal failure, nephrotic oedema or liver cirrhosis contains abnormally high concentrations of mineralocorticoids [4]. In 1953, Simpson identified aldosterone initially called "electrocortin" and he published its structure in 1954 [5]. In 1955, Wettstein synthesised aldosterone.

And so, Conn was well prepared, intellectually speaking, when he admitted the patient to his laboratory on April 27th, 1954. After taking a history, examining the patient and noting hypertension associated with salt and water imbalance (the patient's serum potassium varied between 1.6 and 2.5 mEq/l!) he considered two possibilities: excessive production of aldosterone or a specific renal tubular defect with potassium loss. Through sophisticated clinical and biological investigations, he came to the conclusion that the first possibility was the correct one. *"It is believed that these studies delineate a new clinical syndrome which is designated temporarily as primary aldosteronism. In its fully developed state it is characterized by the presence in the urine of excessive amounts of a sodium-retaining corticoid, by severe hypokalemia, hypernatremia, alkalosis, and a renal tubular defect in the reabsorption of water [...]. The clinical picture consists of intermittent tetany, paresthesia, periodic severe muscular weakness and "paralyses", polyuria and polydipsia, hypertension, and no edema. Of additional interest is the relative lack of important symptomatology at extreme low levels of serum potassium. The syndrome can occur in the absence of any other demonstrable evidence of increased activity of the adrenal cortices"*.

In November 1954, Conn wrote up his work and submitted his paper to the *Journal of Laboratory and Clinical Medicine*, even though his patient had not yet been treated. He concluded that: *"From a therapeutic point of view and in the light of present knowledge, these data indicate that total adrenalectomy followed by substitution therapy should abolish the entire metabolic abnormality. The patient is now in the hospital in preparation for this procedure. We hope to report other studies, as well as the results of adrenalectomy, at a later date"* [6]. The operation was performed in December just in time for Conn to add a small footnote to his paper published in January 1955: *"On Dec. 10, 1954, operation was performed on M.W. A right adrenal cortical tumor, 4 cm in diameter was removed. The left adrenal gland was left in situ. Further studies are now in progress"*.

3. Conn J.W., Louis L.H. Production of endogenous salt-active corticoids as reflected in the concentrations of sodium and chloride of thermal sweat. *J Clin Endocrinol* 1950; 10: 12.

4. On this subject, Conn cited the work of Simpson, Deming, Chart and Singer published between 1950 and 1954.

5. Simpson S.A., Tait J.F., Wettstein A., Neher R., von Euw J., Schindler O., Reichstein T. Die Konstitution des Aldosterons (The structure of aldosterone). *Helv Chim Act* 1954; 37: 1800-1808.

6. What impact did Conn's publications have on cardiology ? It would appear that the relevance of endocrinology was not immediately apparent to cardiologists, if one judges by the fact that between 1955 and 1958, the French journal *Les Archives du coeur, des vaisseaux et du sang* (Archives of the heart, vessels and blood) did not make any mention of Conn's publications.

As emphasised by Levy, chance undoubtedly played a part in saving the patient. Levy's account is interesting and warrants mention [7]: *"To arrest the course of the disease and thereby prevent a fatal outcome, there was only one way: to remove both of the patient's adrenal glands. To compensate for the severe, fatal consequences of this type of operation, he intended to administer replacement therapy by giving daily adrenal gland extracts, including cortisone. This approach can be likened to human experimentation. The very idea of such an operation is frightening. It runs counter to the Hippocratic spirit and offends our sense of medical ethics [8] [...]. It is a fatal operation which could not be undertaken without subsequent daily replacement therapy. But how hazardous is such therapy? The patient's life is constantly in danger, exposed to major general problems, not to mention unforeseen external circumstances which might deny the patient the vital medication.*

The decision was nevertheless taken and the patient was transferred to the surgical ward. In December 1954, Pr. W.J. Braun performed the operation in accordance with Conn's instructions [9]. The surgeon began by making an incision on the right. Why the right? There is no rational explanation, simply a random choice. On uncovering the right adrenal gland, the surgeon was surprised to find a round tumour 4 cm in diameter which he resected, necessarily removing the gland at the same time. Then, following the predefined plan, he made an incision on the left and found a normal adrenal gland which he decided to leave in place contrary to the pre-established plan.

The patient was cured of her hypertension, her salt and water imbalance and hormone problems. The histological examination of the tumour showed that it was an adrenal cortical adenoma. Biological investigations revealed the presence of an extremely large quantity of aldosterone, 75 to 150 times greater than that contained in the porcine adrenal gland. This gives us some idea of the extraordinary degree of abnormal secretion of which the tumour was capable.

This case is undoubtedly of exceptional value not only because of the extremely detailed investigations performed, but also because of the meticulousness and precision with which they were carried out, leading to the conclusion that the clinical symptoms were due to abnormal adrenal function. And one cannot help but wonder what would have happened if the surgeon had started his operation on the left and not on the right. Had this been the case, he no doubt would have followed the pre-established plan and removed the normal adrenal gland on the left. Then, secondarily discovering the tumour on the right he would have been obliged to remove it together with the adrenal gland. In so doing he would have deprived medical science of the absolute proof that the adenoma alone was responsible for the disease and the door would have been left open to all sorts of speculative considerations.

7. Levy A. Le rendez-vous manqué de la connaissance immédiate et du hasard. Contribution à l'histoire de l'hypertension artérielle (The missed rendez-vous between immediate understanding and chance. Contribution to the history of arterial hypertension). *Coeur et médecine interne* 1979; XVIII, n°4: 567-570.

8. In 1942, R. Fontaine was summoned by a professor of medicine to Toulouse to perform a resection of both adrenal glands in a severely hypertensive patient. There was no suspicion of a tumour. Fontaine removed only one of the adrenal glands and performed only a very partial resection on the other. This tells us something about his feelings towards the indication to operate which he considered perilous, possibly even "insane", Levy reports in an oral communication.

9. Conn J.W., Laurence H.L. Primary aldosteronism. A new clinical entity. *Ann Int Med* 1956: 44: 1-15.

Chance, that mysterious and imponderable factor, by guiding the surgeon's hand to the right and not to the left, changed this woman's fate and secured her well-being".

The epilogue is history: medical imaging techniques (initially the retropneumoperitoneum, then arteriography and CAT-scanning) now guide the hand of the surgeon who, more than any other medical practitioner, abhors the unknown.

Clinical observation was an indispensable component in shedding light on the role of the adrenal cortex in the regulation of blood pressure. But Conn's mind was prepared for this discovery and his contribution to medical science confirmed what Trousseau had said a century earlier: *"You see, gentlemen, there is quite a difference between the scientist who observes and the artist who creates"*. (Armand Trousseau. Medical clinic, Hôtel-Dieu hospital. Paris, 1861). In this particular case, the surgical cure of a symptomatic hypersecreting adenoma was virtually an experiment. The history of medicine, and of endocrinology in particular, is punctuated with such situations in which one unusual case has taught us more than a whole series of more common cases. This story can also be seen as a striking illustration of the need for having the laboratory and the hospital ward close to one another. Perhaps the tribute to Conn would be more complete if we were able to cite the name of the doctor who had the presence of mind to refer the patient to Conn's laboratory. The history of medicine, like the history of war, also has its unsung heros. We should erect a monument to the unknown physician to do justice to all those who, anonymously, have advanced the cause of medical science...

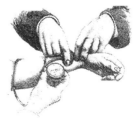

4
TREATING HYPERTENSION

The four periods of antihypertensive treatment

"In an attempt to quieten his patient's agitation, Cottard tried the milk diet. However the endless milk soups had no effect because my grandmother added a great deal of salt to them, and at that time people were unaware of the disadvantages of doing this (Widal not yet having made his discoveries). Medicine being a compendium of successive and conflicting errors by doctors, in summoning the best among them, there is every chance that a truth earnestly sought will be deemed false some years later. So that to believe in medicine would be utter folly, but not to believe in it would be an even greater one, since in the end some truths have emerged from this mass of errors".

Marcel Proust [1]
A la recherche du temps perdu (1913)
(In remembrance of things past)

1. French novelist (1871-1922). Both his father and his brother were physicians. He himself was a severe asthma sufferer. His writings contain a number of references to interesting aspects of early 20th century medicine.

The evolution of antihypertensive therapy is a maze in which one can easily get lost, for medical practice depends on its context in time. One must avoid judging the past from a contemporary angle. For over a century, practitioners have tried to control hypertension by means of surprisingly varied remedies, which often reflected the physiopathological theories of the time. A clinical understanding of hypertension, a knowledge of its physiopathology and the pharmacology regulating arterial pressure are three parameters which, like the planets, have been part of the evolutionary process: they possess trajectories which are both free but also interdependent. In other words, the history of antihypertensive treatment cannot be reduced to a list of therapies. Means cannot be separated from their ends and the rules governing pressure reduction have changed. This chapter should be read in parallel with those dealing with the history of the physiopathology of hypertension and the recognition of vascular risk factors. Looking beyond the bibliographical milestones of the published material, we should also remember that fashion can have an influence. The fascination for a "new" treatment and the heavy legacy of convention have also to be considered. In all disciplines, therapy oscillates between eagerly anticipated innovations and inertia. The treatment of hypertension is no exception.

Bearing these remarks in mind, one can appreciate why an innovative publication on the effects of salt on blood pressure is not synonymous with the introduction of a salt-free diet for hypertensive patients, or that a surgical treatment for hypertension which yesterday was judged as useful is today recognised as useless or dangerous. At any given moment the two types of therapy, the one "modern" and the other "obsolete", can coexist.

In spite of these reservations, we can attempt to distinguish different periods in the history of antihypertensive treatment which we could call the Prehistoric period, the Middle Ages, the Renaissance and the Golden Age. Weaknesses are inherent in divisions of this type, since in medicine, the old does not drive out the new in orderly sequence.

To summarise the history of the therapy of hypertension, it should be remembered that there was no truly effective medical treatment available prior to the Second World War. The Veterans Administration study in 1970 effectively demonstrated the existence of a valid treatment for moderate hypertension [2].

2. Veterans Administration Cooperative Study Group on antihypertensive agents. Effects of treatment on morbidity and mortality in hypertension. II. Results in patients with diastolic blood pressure averaging 90 through 114 mmHg. *JAMA* 1970; 213: 143-152.

This was the first randomised study against placebo showing the benefit of treatment of hypertension in the prevention of cerebral vascular accidents, renal failure, cardiac failure and dissecting aneurysm of the aorta (but not heart attack). It was also demonstrated that treatment prevented progression to severe hypertension. In the United States, the National Blood Pressure Education Program was created at this time and from then on made use of public funds to promote antihypertensive treatment, notably via the media. In 1985, the publication of the results of the MRC Trial in the treatment of mild hypertension [3] confirmed these data but raised the question of the cost-effectiveness of the benefit, which was sometimes minimal, of treating millions of individuals. Other studies, showed that a reduction in the level of blood pressure alone was not sufficient and that the lifestyle of patients, (particularly smoking) and their cholesterol levels also had to be taken into account.

3. Medical Research Council Working Party. MRC Trial of treatment of mild hypertension: principal results. *Br Med J.* 1985; 291: 97-104.

THE PREHISTORIC PERIOD: THE ABSENCE OF METHODOLOGY, EFFECTIVENESS AND OBJECTIVES

By "the prehistoric period" we refer to that period of exploration when doctors advanced through unknown territory with no predetermined route to guide them and with no precise idea even of the goal they were pursuing. This was so for the first pioneers, who made some progress without ever fully outlining their objectives. Until the 1920s, treating raised arterial pressure involved working in an experimental situation with no defined parameters, where physiopathological theories with little if any rational basis were advanced and clinical data were considered in a non-structured manner. Articles or chapters in textbooks entitled

The treatment of arterial hypertension did appear, but even the status of the hypertensive patient was vague, as were the aims of the treating doctor. The clinical circumstances were extremely varied and at times were chosen from very different specialities. Those treating were usually internists, less frequently cardiologists. Nephrology did not exist as a separate medical entity at the time. Treatment objectives were also extremely vague, even sometimes contested. In 1931 certain authors were still writing that raised arterial pressure should not be reduced [4]. This consideration alone well illustrates the complexity surrounding the treatment of hypertension at the time.

For many years, medicine ignored the methodology of evaluation, although it had been theoretically described by the statisticians. Therapeutic modalities were assessed on very small numbers of patients who were rarely comparable and trials against placebo were unheard of. Results were unreliable and were affected by the method of measurement of the blood pressure, which was still in its infancy. The subjectivity of the experimenter compounded his difficulties in the absence of the objectivity afforded by statistical methods. The lack of clarity in this context favoured deadlock (for example whether to treat the symptoms of hypertension or the "arteriosclerosis"). Thus the principles behind dietary salt restriction had been well documented from 1904 onwards by Ambard and Beaujard, but they had not been accepted into clinical practice. This situation was not to change for another forty years. Even worse was that the therapeutic era was initially so confused that it was difficult to distinguish valid science from the offerings of visionaries and charlatans. It should be remembered that the first publication concerning the miraculous effects of insulin in diabetes (1920-1922) met with scepticism from the leading authorities, who remained understandably cautious, tired as they were of hearing the false promises emanating from an unrestrained medical press on an almost daily basis. Irrespective of the intelligence of the reader, it was not easy in the 1920s to separate the wheat from the chaff. And supposing that electrotherapy did reduce blood pressure easily and painlessly? And supposing that irradiation of the adrenals was the best treatment for hypertension? In 1910, these questions were not thought to be ludicrous. Certainly, history judges ideas, but one should exercise caution when assessing them retrospectively.

4. Harris I., Pratt C.L.G. Should high blood pressure be reduced? *Lancet* 1931; 629-630.

THE MIDDLE AGES: EARLY VICTORIES... AT A PRICE.

The Middle Ages followed, and from then on it was easier to surround the enemy, in particular malignant hypertension, with a formidable range of violent but effective weaponry.

Volhard and Fahr described malignant hypertension in 1914 as a disease of renal origin [5]. Hypertensive patients were now reported as suffering from benign or malignant hypertension. Going one step further, Keith and Wagener in 1939 used four categories to study the evolution and prognosis of hypertension [6].

Their publication was an invitation to practitioners to use the classification they recommended so that a common language could be adopted. They argued for an approach based on the clinical degree of severity rather than on an aetiological classification of limited use. At this time the aetiological investigation of hypertension was at a standstill and their viewpoint established a basic precondition for the modern assessment of treatment. But up to the 1950s, whilst publications on the short-term effects of different compounds on blood pressure appeared regularly, there was very little information available on mortality and survival rates [7].

Concern for effective treatment meant that the severely hypertensive patient was faced with an awesome armamentarium. When nitrites and mistletoe powder were no longer effective, the scalpel held sway. More effective than blood-letting, sympathectomy finally achieved reduction in dangerous pressure levels. For the first time, the prognosis for the patient improved. An important objective had been achieved.

Peet, concerned with the differing standards for deciding on treatment, classified his patients according to the severity of their condition in order to judge the results of sympathectomy. He felt that the term "benign hypertension" should be banned, since sooner or later, he claimed, vascular damage would occur [8]. A methodology for assessment was emerging. Patients were selected by a trial and error method, follow-up was pursued for up to twelve years and inclusion-exclusion criteria were defined for more than 1,500 patients. The modern critical approach was essentially in place, although there was still much room for improvement. The goals were now much clearer and sometimes even ambitious. Smithwick noted that one quarter of the adult population was hypertensive and that it was very desirable to reduce the mortality in this condition [7]. In these Middle Ages, with no effective drug therapy, the surgeon's knife reigned supreme.

THE RENAISSANCE:

EFFECTIVE DRUGS SUPPLANT SURGERY

By current standards, the era of effective pharmacological treatment started after World War II. But it was preceded by a long period of pathophysiological research and anarchic commercialisation, belonging

5. Volhard F., Fahr K.T. *Die Brightsche Nierenkrankheit: Klinik Pathologie und Atlas* (Bright's disease of the kidney: pathology, clinical aspects and atlas).1914. Julius Springer, Berlin; 8, p. 292.

6. They found a close correlation with survival (cf page 95). Keith N.M., Wagener H.P.P., Barker N.W. Some different types of essential hypertension: their course and prognosis. *Am J Med Sci* 1939; 197: 332-343.

7. Smithwick R.H. Splanchnicectomy for essential hypertension; results in 1,266 cases. *JAMA* 1953; 152: 1501-1504.

8. Peet M.M. Results of bilateral supradiaphragmatic splanchnicectomy for arterial hypertension. *N Engl J Med* 1947; 236: 270-277.

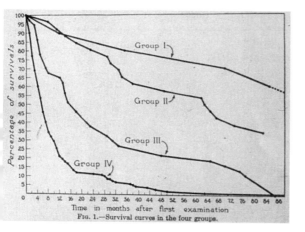

Fig. 1.—Survival curves in the four groups.

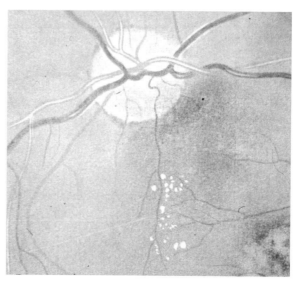

2

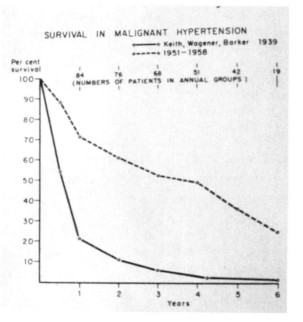

Classification and comparison

In the late 1930s, hypertension was increasingly recognised as an important vascular risk factor, and with the widespread use of pressure measurement, clinicians were well aware of the circumstances of severe hypertension. In spite of this, considerations of prognosis or treatment were vague and the desire to discover the "cause" of hypertension increased the confusion. In 1914, Volhard and Fahr had the merit of clearly distinguishing malignant hypertension through its rapidly dramatic outcome. But apart from these cases, the difficulties inherent in understanding the natural evolution of hypertension made it difficult for various authors to compare their work.

In an article published in the American Journal of Medical Sciences (1939, 197: 332-343) Norman Keith (internist) and Henry Wagener (ophthalmologist) suggested that four groups should be used to classify hypertensive patients: group 1 - few symptoms; group 2 - no retinal signs; group 3 - "moderate vasospastic retinitis"; group 4 - so called "malignant" hypertension.

After following up 200 patients for 5 years, from November 1927 to August 1932, the authors were able to produce survival curves which revealed the gloomy outcome for the pre-war hypertensive patient (*figure 1*). The strength of this study was not so much the intricate histological discussion (their classification was not based on the level of arterial pressure, which was not even mentioned in their article, but on the vascular state of the patients, who had mainly been assessed by fundal examination) (*figure 2*), but rather the fact that it underlined the need for a classification of hypertensive patients, an essential prerequisite for therapeutic studies. In 1958, it was not always possible to produce statistics proving the benefit of blood pressure reduction for the overall population of hypertensive patients (in terms of longevity and reduced incidence of complications). On the other hand, Dustan et al. [12] published the survival curves of subjects suffering from malignant hypertension who had been treated with hexamethonium (responsible for fatal pneumopathy in 8 cases out of 52), chlorisondamine or mecamylamine. The treated group had a 50% mortality rate at 3 years. Although the study is criticisable methodologically, the authors presented their survival curve alongside that of Keith and Wagener, published 20 years earlier (*figure 3*). Some progress had occurred.

to the prehistoric period of hypertensive treatment when there was no clearly effective treatment and when it was impossible to distinguish the promising leads from those with no prospects. In the years from 1910 to 1930, the proponents of the haemodynamic approach praised the merits of the vasodilators (real or supposed), while the endocrinologists, supporters of the adrenal theory of hypertension, were enthused by the hypotensive action of organ extracts.

In the post-war period, a firmer base had been established to justify antihypertensive treatment. By way of sympathectomy, an effective surgical solution had been found for the treatment of malignant hypertension and this in turn stimulated research into ganglion blocking agents capable of inhibiting the sympathetic system. The medical approach appeared to hold promise and occupied the attention of a growing number of researchers. The first effective antihypertensive agent was the antimalarial pentaquine which, in 1946, was recognised to have antihypertensive activity. For the first time, malignant hypertension was improved by medication. Other effective hypotensive agents followed: ganglion blockers, veratrum and rauwolfia alkaloids and vasodilators. Many of these originated in research projects which had been initiated in the early 20th century. However, the incidence of severe side-effects prevented their widespread use, particularly in treating moderate hypertension.

Lyons and his team published a study on the effects of sympathetic blockage with tetraethylammonium and indicated that treatment using the medication repeatedly was not conceivable [9]. Surgical treatment therefore remained very much in use until the end of the 1950s. Brest stated that common hypertension was being neglected or poorly controlled with treatment which was ineffective or outdated [10]. At the other end of the scale, moderate hypertension was also being treated surgically, though the risk/benefit ratio was questionable. The "violence" of the scalpel was still present at a time when the "soft approach" (i.e. effective medication) was making headway.

At the beginning of the 1950s, doctors who had not been won over by the extravagant promises of the medical press were still sceptical about the treatment of hypertension. In 1953, an editorialist from a general medical journal, writing on hypertension explained the situation in these terms: *"A whole issue of this journal would still only have room for the briefest summary of all the miracle drugs for hypertension which, for several decades, have been conceived, brought to life and extolled by the combined fervour of doctors and pharmaceutical companies. Most are scarcely born before they are quickly forgotten — and rightly so. However, despite their total lack of effect on blood pressure, others remain alive for very different and often disconcerting reasons"* [11]. By the 1950s,

9. Lyons R.H. et al. The effects on the autonomic ganglia in man of tetraethylammonium. Preliminary observations on its clinical application. *Am J Med Sci* 1947; 1: 315-323.

10. Brest A.N. Antihypertensive drug therapy: A 30-year retrospective. *Clinical therapeutics* 1992; 14: n°1.

11. Chevalier H. Le traitement de l'hypertension (The treatment of arterial hypertension). *Rev Prat* 1953; 3: n°11. Even today, we know that some of the older treatments have not been removed from the prescriptions. The unsubstantiated concept of "cerebral oxygenating agents" still lives on... the existence of a medication does not only depend on the statistical evidence, it also has to do with the age of the prescribing doctor, that of his patient and with the prevailing legislation (reimbursement, drug surveillance, etc.).

hypertension had acquired the status of a substantial "market", so that, despite their pharmacological inefficacy, a large number of substances were being promoted. On the other hand, patients with hypertension were more and more often being given bad news about their future prospects, due to a better understanding of vascular risk factors. Little wonder that patients anxiously demanded treatment.

The pharmaceutical industry fostered alarmist information about strokes, and also edited "scientific brochures" which it published in the lay press. Anyone could receive, "Free on request", a leaflet on arteriosclerosis and hypertension which inevitably ended by recommending the purchase of a remedy.

Doctors and patients regarded hypertension as a social scourge and impatiently awaited an effective and well-tolerated treatment. In the late 1950s, there was no effective pharmacological solution to the problem of common, moderate hypertension. Dustan et al. [12] made it clear that after long-term drug treatment (a period of 7 or 8 years), there was still no tangible effect on the prevention of the complications of hypertension or on longevity. The use of hexamethonium did have immediate benefits in cases of malignant hypertension. However, the results were neither constant (sometimes there was no response) nor were they easily obtained (there were sometimes extremely serious side-effects such as fatal interstitial pneumopathy), nor were they synonymous with a cure, as the survival curves testify. In their study, 52 of the 84 patients treated had died by seven years from the beginning of treatment (most commonly from cardiac failure). The authors judged this mortality to be "*at first glance discouraging*", but were nevertheless able to show an improvement on comparing their own results with those published 20 years earlier by Keith and Wagener.

In 1958, circumstances were favourable for the appearance of the thiazide diuretics. Epidemiology had produced a better knowledge and understanding of the arterial risk and the surgical experiences and the physiopathological progress had made the benefits of reducing blood pressure clearer. This innovation paved the way for the advent of modern medical treatment. With the arrival of the diuretics, it was now possible to reduce blood pressure in an effective and lasting manner simply by the administration of a tablet with acceptable side-effects. In hypertension, a better treatment than surgery had at long last been discovered. The golden age of pharmacology was about to begin.

12. Dustan H.P., Schneckloth E., Corcoran A.C., Page I.H. The effectiveness of long-term treatment of malignant hypertension. *Circulation* 1958; 18: 644-651.

THE GOLDEN AGE:
NEW PHARMACOLOGICAL CATEGORIES AND
THE ERA OF CONTROLLED TRIALS

The golden age is characterised by effectiveness, abundance and prosperity. Effectiveness for the patient (the era of controlled clinical trials had arrived), abundance for the practitioner (new therapeutic categories enriched his arsenal) and prosperity for the pharmaceutical industry (with cardiovascular drugs the economic stakes were high).

For the three decades from 1960 to 1990, medical research offered doctors new compounds which were effective and complementary, and which at last had been evaluated in statistically mature clinical trials (randomised, large scale, placebo, etc.). The benefit of treating mild to moderate hypertension remained under discussion. At the start of the 1960s, there were no convincing results to support such treatment and there was much controversy [13]. However, in 1963, the Veterans' study commenced under Freis' direction. One hundred and forty-three men (women were not included in the study) with a diastolic pressure ranging from 115 to 129 mm of mercury, received either placebo, or antihypertensive treatment (hydrochlorothiazide, reserpine, hydralazine). In 1967, it was definitively demonstrated, using sound methodology, that the treatment of moderate to moderately severe hypertension had produced a significant benefit [14]. A page had been turned and from then on the ethics of placebo-controlled trials in hypertension were seriously questioned.

With the advent of the diuretics and then the betablockers, the calcium inhibitors and finally the converting enzyme inhibitors, the medical arsenal made control of the majority of patients with essential hypertension possible. It was found that even asymptomatic moderate hypertension could benefit from treatment. This progress in treatment had a noticeable impact on the morbidity of hypertensive patients and during these years the benefit for patients was proved beyond doubt by strict methodological criteria. The dramatic situation of malignant hypertension became increasingly rare, while age-related vascular problems took over from hypertension, which was no longer the only risk factor to be considered.

In 1971, the Albert Lasker prize was awarded to Edward Freis of the Veterans Administration for *"demonstrating the effectiveness of drug treatment in hypertension; demonstrating the value of medication in preserving life, even in mild hypertension; and demonstrating the reduction in deaths by cerebrovascular accident and congestive cardiac failure, obtained when arterial pressure is reduced to normal values"* [15]. The use of drugs in the treatment of hypertension had been officially acknowledged, a testimony to its importance for society.

13. Perera G.A. Antihypertensive drug versus symptomatic treatment in primary hypertension: effect on survival. *JAMA* 1960; 173: 11-13

14. Veterans Administration Cooperative Study Group on anti-hypertensive agents. Effects of treatment on morbidity in hypertension. *JAMA* 1967; 202: 116-122.

15. Cited by K. Beyer Jr. *Discovery of Thiazides. Perspectives in Biology and Medicine.* Springer 1977; 20: 410-420.

In 1988, it was the turn of the Nobel prize for medicine to celebrate this victory against hypertension in its award to Sir James Black who, according to the description of the Nobel committee, "*has grasped the great pharmacological possibilities offered by the medications known as receptor blocking agents and who, in 1964, developed the first betablocking drug, propranolol*".

AN UNCERTAIN FUTURE

In the prevention of cardiovascular disease, the most spectacular results on mortality and morbidity are without doubt behind us, since in the industrialised countries with a good health care system, severely hypertensive patients are in the main detected and treated. Even though there is always room for improvement, the reduction in vascular risk through lowering of blood pressure has been, in large part, achieved. Even if more effective antihypertensive compounds were to become available in the near future, they would probably not have any determinant effect on mortality or morbidity. The enemy today is no longer arterial pressure taken in isolation, but rather a collection of several factors among which age is the most important. A page has been turned.

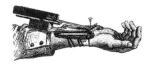

An assorted catalogue of treatments:
Radiotherapy, electrotherapy,
pyrotherapy, surgery and pharmacology

"Treatment inevitably conveys hope, if not fear, transforming the desire to help into reality. This single reason causes it to lose clearness and we become unable to define it in absolutely precise terms. The power of the doctor and the trust of the patient mingle with its cold and characterless substance".

François Dagonet
La Raison et les Remèdes (Reason and Remedies).
Presses Universitaires de France, Paris. 1984.

The following is an incomplete catalogue of the main types of hypertensive treatment. For each one, the aim is to follow a chronological pattern, but as we have indicated previously, the history of these types of therapy is interlinked. Equally, we should have specified whether these methods referred to severe or mild cases of hypertension, and whether they related to secondary or essential hypertension. This was not possible since such distinctions were not clearly made in the past. We have decided to elaborate on the history of darsonvalisation radiotherapy and pyrotherapy, areas in the history of hypertension which are little known. These techniques are certainly somewhat anecdotal, but they illustrate the degree of indecision which prevailed in the first half of the 20th century. The history of a subject should not just be about events validated by history but should also relate the setbacks. The account which follows does not claim to be exhaustive, and notably the numerous compounds which preceded the diuretics are missing [1].

BLOOD-LETTING AND ANTI-APOPLECTIC ELIXIR: THE TIME OF HELPLESSNESS

In the Sainte-Agnès ward of the Hôtel-Dieu hospital in Paris on March 3rd 1856, Geneviève B. had been stricken with apoplexy for 48 hours. Her arm was gradually coming back to life and she appeared to be more alert. Leeches applied to the cervical region, produced a large degree of blood-letting and had allowed her to avoid the worst. In spite of being hypertrophied, the heart of this patient with albuminuria was holding up well and she was less breathless. Her pulse, which when

1. Hines E.A. Thiocyanate in the treatment of hypertensive disease. *Med Clin N Am* 1946; 30: 869-877.
Burt C.C, Graham A.J.P. Pentamethonium iodide in the investigation of peripheral vascular disease and hypertension. *Br Med J* 1950; 1: 455-460.
Krayer O. The pharmacology of the veratrum alkaloids. *Physiol Rev* 1946; 26: 383-446.
Cohn J.N. Haemodynamic effects of guanethidine in man. *Circ Res* 1963; 12: 298-307.

palpated initially was quite feeble, had strengthened, a good prognostic sign, although clinical examination of her arteries revealed a generalised arteriosclerosis which for a 43-year-old woman was very early, doubtless due to alcohol and hereditary syphilis. Bed rest and a strict diet consisting solely of milk would take care of the rest. Had the leeches greatly influenced this improvement? Broussais was convinced that they had, but Pierre Louis was more sceptical. This pioneer of the numerate method thought that the answer would only be apparent once the failures and therapeutic successes had been strictly assessed. Did anyone have the right to evaluate the master's teaching in such a way? This was 19th century France and the answer was "no" [2].

In spite of the predominance of a mortality and morbidity of infectious origin, the hospital admitted an increasing number of cases with apoplexy and angina. These diseases were not rare and their association with changes in the cerebral or coronary circulation was often confirmed at autopsy. The disease was therefore arterial, but in other cases the kidney appeared to be a causal factor, as Richard Bright had demonstrated in patients with albuminuria. Specific treatments were limited: the therapeutic arsenal consisted of opium, digitalis, blood-letting, amyl nitrite and diets. Naturally, hypertension was absent from the pathophysiological discussion which concentrated basically on cardiac or renal insufficiency and the degeneration of the vessels. Hypertension would have to wait for the new ideas of Traube, Marey, Basch and Potain before appearing, and even then, it was misunderstood in the clinical setting. By the end of the 19th century, the large textbooks included chapters on "hypertrophy of the heart, angina pectoris, adipose overload of the heart, bradycardias and tachycardias, palpitations and aortitis", but on hypertension as an illness — nothing. However, when an elevation in arterial pressure was cited, as in the *Treatise of applied therapeutics* by Albert Robin, in which the section on cardiology was compiled in collaboration with Huchard, there was constant reference to a link with arteriosclerosis. "*Almost all patients with angina have hypertension, which initially precedes and then accompanies the development of arteriosclerosis and for which the primary therapeutic indication is to use health measures and medication to combat the tendency to hypertension*" [3]. This was certainly an innovative phrase but not in the sense in which we understand hypertension today. Hypertension had not yet gained the status of a disease. In 1913, it was still the case that hypertension and arteriosclerosis were considered one and the same. The textbooks asserted that "*it is very difficult to study medication for hypertension without constantly encroaching on the subject of therapy for arteriosclerosis*" and they concluded that preventive treatment for hypertension "*is the same as that of early arteriosclerosis*" [4].

This assimilation explains why the history of the treatment of elevated arterial pressure began even before hypertension was defined as a modern

2. See the note about the numerate method in chapter 2 — Recognising hypertension.

3. Robin A., Huchard H. Part XI, *Traitement des maladies de l'appareil circulatoire* (Treatment of diseases of the circulation). Paris. 1897.

4. Gilbert A., Carnot P. *Médications symptomatiques, circulatoires, hématiques et nerveuses* (Symptomatic, circulatory, haematic and nervous medications). 1913, Baillière. Paris, p. 136.

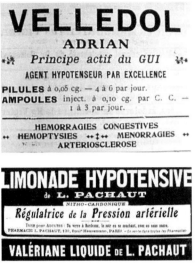

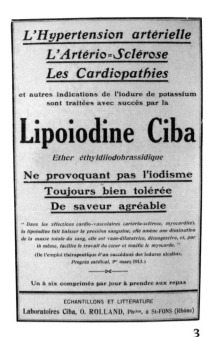

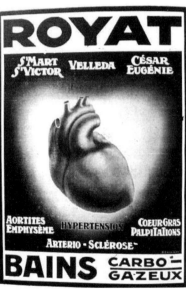

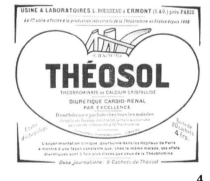

3

4

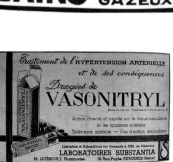

Numerous forgotten remedies.

Current antihypertensive agents are so effective that yesterday's drugs have been forgotten. Although the tablets, ampoules, mixtures and various preparations prescribed for hypertension were no doubt ineffective, they flourished in the early 20th century. A look at the advertisements published between 1912 and 1917 in the Archives of the heart, vessels and blood bear witness to this fact.

"Velledol Adrian", "*hypotensive agent par excellence*" was widely used for arteriosclerosis, congestive haemorrhages and haemoptyses (*figure 1*).

L. Pachaut's "hypotensive lemonade" was "*a regulator of arterial pressure*". The recommended adult dose was "*a wine glassful, with or without sugar on retiring to bed*" (*figure 2*).

Iodised products such as "Lipoiodine Ciba" were unequalled in "*reducing arterial pressure, reducing total blood mass, being vasodilatory and decongestive and by the same token assisting the effort of the heart and toning up the myocardium*" (*figure 3*).

"Theosol", "*a cardio-renal diuretic par excellence*", had the advantage (significant in 1917!) of "*having no similarity with the German theobromine pseudo-salts*" (*figure 4*). Finally should any of these products fail, a stay at Royat spa was definitely indicated. Its "*carbo-gaseous baths*" would surely be effective in "*aortitis, emphysema, fatty heart, arteriosclerosis and hypertension*" (*figure 5*). Nitrate derivatives were proposed by Huchard as early as the end of the 19th century (*figure 6*).

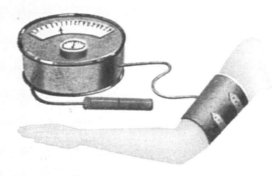

Advertisement from the French medical press in the 1950s

The advertisement reads: "A NEW INDICATION: sodium thiosulfate blocks hypertensive phenylamines such as thyramine, rids the liver of arylated toxic substances and stimulates the metabolism of vascular walls — LONG-TERM TREATMENT OF HYPERTENSION.

entity. The attitudes of doctors were guided by the anatomico-clinical views of arteriosclerosis. If effective remedies were very rare, medical advice was in abundance. Fencing, bicycling, horse-riding, cold baths, staying by the seaside or in the mountains were forbidden for patients with arteriosclerosis. They were, on the other hand encouraged to purify themselves with spa cures. In case one should think otherwise, the lack of pharmacological effectiveness of the old remedies did not imply that therapy should be withheld. Far from it!

THE EXTRAVAGANT PROMISES OF ELECTROTHERAPY: HYPERTENSIVE PATIENTS CONFINED IN CAGES

Doctors, as in the population at large, include individuals who are conservative and therefore hostile to innovations and others who are more inclined to adopt a modern approach. For "progressive" therapists, enthusiasm was justified by the novelty of the approach, since basically this implied a novel effectiveness. And what was valid in the realm of mechanics, home appliances, chemistry or agriculture had to apply to medicine: newly invented methods and appliances aroused hopes where subjectivity abounded. The fact that something was new was as good as a pathological justification!

The use of x-rays and electricity in medicine was of this sort of innovation, by doctors dabbling in physics. It is no surprise to find that hypertension was included in the long list of pathologies which the inventions of the century claimed to have conquered . In this context, the history of the treatment of hypertension offers us several prime examples of medical fantasy. A fantasy which originated in the credulity of some and ended in iatrogenic effects for others. The pursuit of progress brought together engineers, doctors and patients, encouraged by the manufacturers of medical equipment, only too eager to sell their gadgets such as the electric belt, sold in the 1890s and claim to cure all ills, including impotence. The growing fascination with the magic of electricity was such that claims for these multiple benefits were readily accepted without any objective evaluation.

In the treatment of hypertension the period between 1890 and 1920 was particularly confused as the concept of hypertension was new and as yet not well established. Equally, the long tradition of atherosclerosis with its multiple therapies was at the forefront of the discussion. However, popularity or originality were not synonymous with success. The use of electricity and x-rays in the treatment of hypertension represents a little-known page in the history of medicine and demonstrates how reputable scientists were hardly distinguishable from the eccentrics and the visionaires.

The history of medical electricity dates back to antiquity if we are to believe the Greek texts which describe several observations made by doctors on the torpedo ray fish. However it was not until the 18th century that a truly scientific approach began with the discovery of electrochemical phenomena, and this rapidly entered the electrotherapy scene [5]. At the end of the 19th century, the fascination with electrotherapy was on the increase. There was some promising research performed, like that into cardiac stimulation or the electric scalpel, while other lines of research led to nothing. Such was the case in hypertension with darsonvalisation.

Darsonvalisation [6], named after its inventor Professor Arsène d'Arsonval (1851-1940), consisted in the application of high frequency currents to the body. During the winter of 1890-1891, in his lectures at the Collège de France, d'Arsonval publicised his initial results. In the United States in 1891, Tesla was following the same line of approach. In France Dr Moutier, one of the main proponents of the method, described its advantages at the Congress for the advancement of science (Grenoble, 1894). Unlike low frequency currents, the method "*does not produce the phenomenon of tetany*". According to a brochure produced by the manufacturer Radiguet, darsonvalisation "*offers experimental physiology a field of research of the utmost importance and provides medicine with a new curative method of treatment*" [7]. In fact, almost all types of acute and chronic illnesses became indications for electrotherapy. Initially the clinics, and then the doctors' surgeries became equipped with the new apparatus. Although quantification was difficult, the fascination for the process was real and favourable reports were relayed by the popular and medical press. D'Arsonval stated in 1882: "*I am convinced that future therapy will only use curative agents which cause physical changes (heat, light, electricity or other currently unknown agents), that is to say agents travelling through the body without ever remaining in it*" [8].

He made it clear that this "*electrifying process produces no sensation whatever, although its action is very energetic*". Electrotherapy had numerous actions, such as "*the extraordinary activity which it has on nutritional exchanges and on cell life... the increase in heat emitted by the body*", the excitation of the "*vasomotor nervous*" system, "*the hyperactivation of vital functions*" or even "*the reduction in the effects of microbial toxins*". Dithyrambic pseudo-statistics were produced by the "electrotherapy institutes" and the innocuous nature (which is true) of the method was praised. Patients flocked to the surgeries equipped with electrotherapy as if attracted by a magnet. Doctors saw it as a new way of attracting clients. At one time even Sigmund Freud succumbed to the fashion, but disappointed, he soon abandoned it. In this context, where the influence of social pressures weighed more heavily than scientific objectivity, hypertension and arteriosclerosis became indications for darsonvalisation which found its way into the private surgeries and clinics more readily than into the medical schools.

5. In Montpellier in 1749, a work had already been published on the treatment of hemiplegia (Dissertatio medica. De hemiplegia per electricitatem curanda). With the contributions of Galvani, the abbot Nollet, Benjamin Franklin, Volta and Duchenne de Boulogne, the method had evolved and in France in 1857, a specialist journal entitled *Medical Electricity* was published.

6. Originally written d'Arsonvalisation, it later became darsonvalisation — a spelling we have adopted throughout.

7. He even travelled to Quebec to promote electrotherapy.

8. Quoted by Huard. L'évolution de l'électrodiagnostic et de l'électrothérapie (The evolution of electrodiagnosis and of electrotherapy). *Bulletin d'histoire de l'électricité*, vol. 2, December 1983, p. 49.

Historically, it is difficult to determine with certainty who actually first proposed applying high frequency currents to patients with hypertension. In 1905, Augustin Challamel, who wrote his thesis on *Darsonvalisation in arterial hypertension* (Paris, 1905), described the contribution made by Dr Moutier in the field of hypotension and hypertension. Arsène d'Arsonval, former assistant to Claude Bernard, friend of Marey and successor of Brown-Séquard at the Collège de France no doubt thought about this indication himself, but was scarcely involved in clinical medicine. In 1896, d'Arsonval published some observations supporting the success of his method in lowering the blood pressure of three patients (two diabetics and one obese patient). A report in 1897 indicated that in the dog, darsonvalisation caused a reduction in arterial pressure by several centimetres. In 1903, a paper on the subject was presented to the Academy of Sciences. Challamel himself presented a paper to the Academy on February 13th and 27th 1905 and according to him, successes were *"self-evident"* [9].

The high frequency currents were administered by means of solenoids arranged in a *"self-conducting cage"* or in a *"condenser bed"*. The treatment consisted of a *"negative static bath"* for a period of 5 to 20 minutes. The patient sat on a glass-footed stool connected by metal to the negative pole of the static machine, i.e. the solenoid, surrounded by electric wires inside a sort of therapeutic cage. Challamel reported his experiment as follows: *"We placed a patient in the cage after taking his blood pressure. We got him to put his arm between two of the spirals of the cage and rest it on a table placed to the side. We attached a transmitting sphygmograph connected to a controlling drum.... Once a resting trace had been taken for 1 to 2 minutes, we switched on the current, without interrupting the recording. After 5 to 6 minutes, the current was switched off. The experiment was stopped, all the phases having been recorded"*. Although Challamel was conversant with the Riva-Rocci apparatus, he had no personal experience of it and consequently used the Verdin, Potain and Gaertner devices. In his thesis he recorded in detail several pages of assessment on the practical usage and usefulness of the devices. The remarks were fully representative of the discussions of the time concerning the methods of measurement. In France, Potain's apparatus was the principal one used and the *"coefficient of personal error"* involved was indicated as being *"not negligible"*.

Success was of course assured, as in all cases with this sort of treatment, dominated by the prevailing ideologies. In 1904, Dr Moutier himself obtained promising results. *"Currently, there can be no further doubt about the action of darsonvalisation, given that through the use of a sphygmometer or a sphygmomanometer, reductions in the blood pressure of hypertensive patients can be recorded after each session in conditions such that the observed results cannot be ascribed to errors of measurement. At the start of treatment, in the first session, we observe*

9. Challamel A. Etude comparative sur l'action de la cage auto-conductrice et du lit condensateur dans le traitement de l'hypertension artérielle par la darsonvalisation (Comparative study on the action of the self-conducting cage and the condenser bed in the treatment of arterial hypertension by darsonvalisation). *Académie des Sciences*, February 13th and 27th 1905.

falls in pressure of 3, 4, 5 and even 6 cm of mercury in the space of a few minutes". A little further on the author added that *"in the final sessions, the reductions in pressure are less considerable"*. After having treated 50 patients, Challamel, now working with Moutier, indicated that *"in patients presenting with permanent severe hypertension, the arterial pressure returned to normal in less than three sessions in the majority of cases"* [10]. Quite convincing proof!

Did these results, obtained through the use of a method which we know today to be totally ineffective, involve deceit? The answer can be found by reading between the lines of a commentary by Moutier: *"The action of darsonvalisation is very rapid. In the cases we have studied, an effect is seen within a minute or two of starting the session. The maximum effect is achieved within two to five minutes, and we have never obtained a greater reduction by prolonging the session"*. It is probable that the observed fall in pressure was due to the effects of rest, which were known and had been described in 1905. However, in their enthusiasm, the authors disregarded any considerations of methodology. Their good faith is not in question, otherwise why would they have published this detail? Their credulity is good testimony to the existence of a medical fantasy world where, regardless of time and place, the constant factor is the subjectivity of the researcher. Even more beneficially, Challamel indicated that the lowered pressure was maintained *"after several weeks"*. Moutier reported in 1904 that *"we have looked for cases of hypertension resistant to this method, but we have been unable to find any. Perhaps some will be observed in the future. Sometimes, if we have not obtained the desired result, this was due to a technical or apparatus fault"*. From fantasy we move into the realms of blindness...

In the prevailing climate of enthusiasm, the theories started. In order to explain the effect of high frequency currents on blood pressure, Challamel "demonstrated" that the reduction in pressure brought about by darsonvalisation was accompanied by an elevation in the "arterio-capillary pressure" measured with Gaertner's tonometer. Challamel explained that darsonvalisation *"reversed the arteriolar spasm by reducing the sympathetic tone causing hypertension"*. The author added that this interpretation concurred with d'Arsonval's observations that the ears of rabbits in the induction cage vasodilate. The patient in this way "relaxed".

There were other interpretations of the vasomotor effects of darsonvalisation. Lemoine indicated, during the session of November 28th, 1910 of the Academy of Sciences, that high frequency currents *"lower arterial pressure by promoting the elimination of cholesterine compounds through the urine"*. However, from 1905 onwards, Widal and Vaquez voiced doubts about the validity of the method before the

10. Moutier and Challamel. "Sur 50 nouveaux cas d'hypertension artérielle traitée par la darsonvalisation" (Fifty new cases of arterial hypertension treated with darsonvalisation). Congrès Français de Médecine 7e session, Paris 1904. *Annales d'électrobiologie et de radiologie*, Nov. 1904.

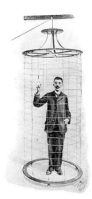

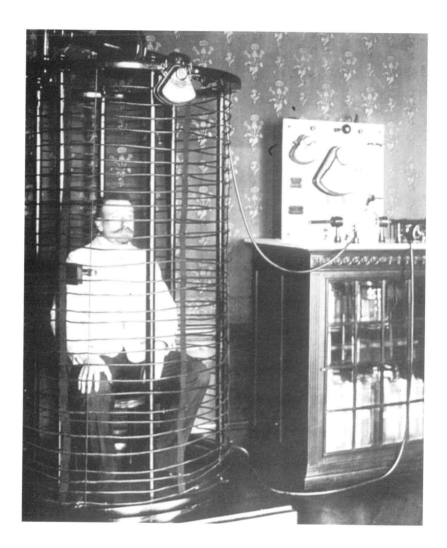

The time of empiricism and credulity: electrotherapy

In vogue at the start of the 20th century, electrotherapy was proposed as a treatment for hypertension. It consisted of "*baths of high frequency current*" delivered by the darsonvalisation process. A paper presented to the Academy of Sciences in 1905 praised its merits:

"*We placed a patient in the cage once his arterial pressure had been taken. We got him to put his arm between two of the spirals of the cage and rest it on a table placed to the side. We attached a transmitting sphygmograph...The arterial pressure of patients presenting with permanent hypertension returned to normal in less than 3 sessions in the majority of cases*". The supporters of this method made their claims at a time when therapeutic trials using proper methodology did not exist.

French Association for the Advancement of Science. In fact, the opinions voiced were contradictory and some began to challenge electrotherapy as a method which thrived on credulity or smacked of charlatanism.

Once the enthusiasm had waned, Gilbert's treatise on therapeutics in 1913 attempted to clarify the situation, although it must be said not entirely with success. *"Let us come now to a method of treatment on which great hopes have been built and which, its enthusiasts claim, has a direct and marvellous action on hypertension: I am referring to darsonvalisation.*

It is difficult to form an opinion about the effects of sinusoidal currents on the symptoms of hypertension. There is a lack of consensus amongst doctors who deal specifically with electricity. We recall Moutier's results, obtained with patients in the Nanterre asylum and how he observed that levels of blood pressures which had reached 18 to 29 centimetres (Potain's apparatus) fell to normal within the space of a single session. It is interesting to compare these results with the rather disappointing observations of Delherm and Laguerrière, who recorded only inconstant and minor changes in pressure. Their observations were substantiated by the results of Bergognié, Broca and Ferrié, based on 39 cases studied under strict scientific conditions. They concluded that d'Arsonval's currents had no effect on blood pressure [...] How can the clinician, confused by these contradictory reports, form a valid opinion on the true merits of the method? In my opinion, the answer might lie in some of the observations made by the supporters of the method themselves. Moutier, when comparing patients from the Nanterre institute with patients from his own private practice, noted that with the latter, 6 to 10 sessions were needed to obtain the same results as could be obtained with one session in the former group.

He attributed this to the fact that patients from his private practice were on a less strenuous diet than those from the asylum. Lately, some of the supporters of darsonvalisation have located their successfully treated patients of the previous 2, 3 and even 5 years and examined them in order to find out what had happened to their blood pressure. Some of the subjects were found to have maintained a low blood pressure whilst others were found to be suffering from their previous, or even higher levels of hypertension. The first group had remained on the diet they had been given, while the others had abandoned it or were once again subject to physical and mental stresses. Perhaps the logical conclusion one can draw from these observations is that the doctor who does not use solenoids may find consolation in the fact that in the end it is diet which is important and that depending on how strict it is, it will have a greater or lesser influence on the effects of sinusoidal currents".

This judgement illustrates just how far the idea of controlled trials for hypertension was from being accepted... In 1931, Riesman [11] indicated in an article in the JAMA that he was still undecided about the advantages of electrotherapy and left his options open: "*High frequency currents appear to be able to reduce blood pressure. My experience is that this effect is not permanent. However there are some proponents of electrotherapy who claim to have obtained lasting results. I have not observed this*". On the eve of the Second World War, darsonvalisation was still accorded some mention in the literature. Sometimes referred to as "diathermy", the method was not totally abandoned. Dumas, without specifying more fully, indicated that "*in the hands of experienced technicians it can produce effective results*", proof of the lack of objectivity, methodology and understanding at that time [12].

11. Riesman D. High blood pressure and longevity. *JAMA* April 4, 1931.

RADIOTHERAPY: "A RATIONAL THERAPEUTIC APPROACH AIMED AT THE CAUSE OF HYPERTENSION"

X-rays were discovered by Röntgen exactly a century ago and were adopted into medical practice remarkably quickly, revolutionising investigational methods and therapeutics. At the beginning of the 20th century x-rays sucessfully gave rise to the techniques of radiology and radiotherapy. Their success is still unchallenged, with many new applications today.

The sensitivity of living tissues to x-rays was evident from the time of their discovery and permitted the development of new types of therapy, notably against cancer. However the fascination with radium and x-rays, which was largely shared by the public, initially concealed the risks inherent in their handling. Awareness of the dangers of ionising radiation came later and in the meantime, the prevailing optimism led to x-rays being tried in many fields such as in hyperhidrosis by the destruction of the sweat glands, in acne through the application of x-rays to the face or even in pediculosis by irradiating the whole body. The initial indications for radiotherapy were eclectic and included endocrine tumours, which had recently been discovered. In Germany in 1904, the first trials on the adrenal glands in Addison's disease were undertaken and in a thesis on the action of x-rays on the adrenal glands [Paris 1913], Paul-Henri Cottenot emphasised that "*no-one has used this agent, which regulates glandular secretion, to reduce the excessive function of the hyperplastic adrenals. And yet modern concepts tell us how important this adrenal hyperplasia is in vascular pathology. Many people believe it to be the essential factor in vascular hypertension and atheroma*". With this concept, the proposal to use irradiation of the adrenals as a hypotensive treatment was made. The young Cottenot, working under the direction of Professors Zimmern and Mulon, explained that "*by introducing this therapy for hypertension, the value of which will only be known in the future, we are convinced that we*

12. Dumas A. *La Maladie hypertensive*. 1939. Masson. Paris.

are providing a new argument supporting theories that are still disputed". He ended by stating that "*the results we have obtained through irradiation of the adrenals of hypertensive patients support this viewpoint*".

Cottenot irradiated 28 "permanently hypertensive" patients and divided them into four groups as follows: "hypertensive patients with no albuminuria; arteriosclerotic patients with no albuminuria; hypertensive patients with albuminuria and arteriosclerotic patients with albuminuria".

For the irradiation, the patient was seated and the 12th rib located. The operator traced a circular outline of the adrenals with a pencil and irradiated each in succession, protecting the spinal cord with a strip of lead. The sessions were subsequently repeated "*depending on the need, as frequently as possible without causing a radiodermatitis*". The arterial pressure was monitored during this process of irradiation using the Pachon and Vaquez devices. Systolic variations alone were assessed since in 1913 the measurement and interpretation of the diastolic pressure was still poorly established. In the absence of a defined protocol, blood pressure was checked weekly for approximately four months. Cottenot's thesis included observations on 29 subjects. "*Treatment with radiotherapy resulted in the reduction of arterial pressure in our patients. It was shown to be effective in the vast majority of cases as out of 29 subjects treated, only 4, who had experienced a small and transient improvement, were found to have a pressure which returned to its original level, where it remained despite repeated irradiation. The duration of the period of reduction in blood pressure is very variable. In some subjects it persists for more than six months, while from time to time in others, it is necessary to treat the rise in blood pressure with new episodes of irradiation. Accompanying the reduction in pressure, the subjects treated experience an improvement in the functional symptoms caused by hypertension; at least this is what we observed in the majority of cases*".

In conclusion, Cottenot saw suprarenal irradiation as being a "*rational therapy, since it addresses the actual cause of the functional problem*". Those operators using the technique sought to justify the effects of their machine through their own interpretation of the pathophysiology of hypertension, much in the same way as those who used electrotherapy. From a disease which was due to "arterial spasm" in the context of darsonvalisation, hypertension became an "adrenal pathology" in the context of radiotherapy. These similarities illustrate how, in the field of medical experimentation, the ideas of the researcher can be adapted to suit the facts. Moreover, the facts can be distorted to suit the theory. The following account of the history of irradiation of the sympathetic region or the carotid sinus is another illustration of the influence of ideological factors in the history of medicine.

In the years from 1920 to 1930, irradiation of almost any part of the body was used to reduce the pressure of hypertensive patients. In addition to the adrenals, the pituitary gland, the neck, the temporal region and even the spine were irradiated. The results published were often encouraging, although the animal experiments appeared less convincing. In 1922, attention was even drawn to the fact that patients who had undergone *"extensive and profound irradiation"* of 20 to 30 hours duration, developed a *"sudden fall in pressure with tachyarhythmia"* [13] due to the effect on the blood pressure of irradiation of the carotid sinuses. There appeared to be *"a relationship between the dose received and the degree of pressure reduction obtained, irrespective of any important digestive or haematological changes"* [14]. In France, as well as in Spain, America or Germany, the manometer had appeared in the radiotherapy ward [15].

Irradiation of the carotid sinus appeared to be physiologically logical and *"its usefulness in the treatment of hypertension must be acknowledged"*, Dooren and Melot affirmed in 1938, and added that *"whatever the outcome of the method, we concur with the observations of the Spanish authors that a hypertensive patient who has been irradiated always experiences a subjective degree of euphoria which is real and variable. These are grounds for considering the use of irradiation in the chronically hypertensive patient in whom all other treatments produce fatigue or affect nutrition"*. It is clear that in the treatment of hypertension, what we call "the prehistoric period", and by this we mean subjectivity and medically ineffective treatment, still existed at the start of the 1940s.

In 1939, irradiation of the adrenals was still included by Dumas among the range of antihypertensive treatments: *"Very precise statistics reported by Langeron and Desplats, cite some favourable cases, some setbacks and some mediocre results"* [16]. The era of unrestrained enthusiasm for radiotherapy was coming to an end but even so, very little mention was made of its harmful effects, as was also the case in other circumstances...

FROM PYROGENS TO HEAT SHOCK GENES

At a time when only "rice diet" and the surgical inhibition of sympathetic nervous systems were unpleasant or uncomfortable therapeutic options in severe hypertension, one particular pioneering approach received attention: "Pyrotherapy". A concept well developed in the 1930's, it was based on the notion of *Febris salutaris*, a beneficial effect of fever. Initially applied in the control of infection or inflammatory processes (syphilis, gonorrhoea, poliomyelitis, multiple sclerosis), it generally used infectious agents (paludism) or protein extracts (kidney homogenates) but also external heat (infrared radiation) to increase body temperature. Early on, the cardiovascular consequences of pyrotherapy

13. Coutard and Lavedan, cited by F.V. Dooren and G. Melot.

14. Dooren F.V., Melot G. Effet de l'irradiation des sinus carotidiens sur la tension artérielle. (The effect on the blood pressure of carotid sinuse irradiation). *Archives du coeur et des vaisseaux*. 1938; 1: 178-203.

15. For further details, see the bibliography quoted by Dooren.

16. Dumas A. *La maladie hypertensive* (Hypertensive disease) ibid.

were recognised. Both French and American authors of that time suggested limited "therapeutic sessions" of pyrexia below a pulse rate of 160. It was realised that blood pressure increased early in the therapy followed by its decrease. An increase followed by a decrease of pulse pressure was also described, together with capillary vasoconstriction followed by vasodilation [17].

Already at that time, Halphen and Auclair (cited by Richet [17]) realised that the blood pressure decline was accentuated in hypertensive patients and persisted for weeks to several months. Together with the decrease of blood pressure, Laubry [18] observed relief of symptoms (headaches, dizziness). In addition to lowering blood pressure in hypertensives, pyrotherapy was used with "success" in the peripheral artery obstructive disease acrocyanosis or Raynaud's disease, and even in angina.

The most convincing description and study of the benefits of pyrogen therapy are owed to Irvine H. Page. With Robert D. Taylor, he developed this treatment, particularly for malignant hypertension, at the Cleveland Clinic in Ohio [19]. Page reported the use of kidney extracts and Baxter's soluble bacterial pyrogen (Pyromen) in 20 patients with malignant hypertension. The therapy was administered 5 days per week to cause an increase of temperature to 42°C. Patients were selected to avoid those with advanced renal failure. After "a few weeks of therapy", the benefit lasted for 3 to 6 months or more. First, improvement was seen in the retina. In his early textbook, Page actually documented the disappearance of exudates and haemorrhages by fundi photographs (see figure p. 116) [20]. Although early on salicylates were given to those feeling uncomfortable, it was later realised that the increase in body temperature was indeed required for therapeutic benefit to be fully apparent. Three out of five patients who discontinued the therapy died early of cerebrovascular accidents. A total of 13 patients survived for an average of 32 months and none died of renal failure, although this was the usual fate of untreated malignant hypertensives.

When asked in 1988 about later developments, Page wrote that *"unfortunately no further developments occurred in this area since the invention of pharmacotherapy"* (personal correspondence).

In our current era, half a century later, all pyrogens used are recognised as inducers of heat shock genes (HSPs) in all living organisms, upon stimulation by adverse environments, heat, toxins, heavy metals, alcohol, but also by immobilisation stress, catecholamines, etc. Genetically-defined models of rodent hypertension respond excessively to environmental stress and this property segregates as a distinct genetic locus (tms) of about 15 mmHg [21]. Chronic administration of heat, similarly to the seminal observations of Richet and Page, decreases blood pressure in genetically hypertensive mice [22]. Environmental stress induces several HSPs [23] in cardiovascular tissues in vivo, and this phenomenon is again exaggerated in hypertensive animals [24] as well as in humans [25].

17. Richet C., Surmont J. and Le Gô P. Pyrothérapie (pyrotherapy), 1938, Masson, Librairie de l'Académie de Médecine, Paris.

18. Laubry quoted in Richet C. et al. ibid.

19. Page I.H. and Taylor R.D. Pyrogens in the treatment of malignant hypertension. In: *Modern Concepts of Cardiovascular Disease*, American Heart Association, Vol. XVIII, No. 10, October, 1949.

20. *Arterial Hypertension: Its Diagnosis and Treatment*, Second Edition, Irvine H. Page and Arthur C. Corcoran, Eds., 1949. Year Book Inc.

21. Malo D., Schlager G., Tremblay J. and Hamet P. Thermosensitivity, a possible new locus involved in genetic hypertension. *Hypertension* 1989; 14: 121-128.

22. Malo D., Pang S.C., Schlager G., Tremblay J. and Hamet P. Decrease of blood pressure in spontaneously hypertensive mice by heat treatment. *Am J Hypertens* 1990; 3: 400-404.

23. Udelsman R., Blake M.J., Stagg C.A., Li D.G., Putney D.J. and Holbrook N.J. Vascular heat shock protein expression in response to stress. Endocrine and autonomic regulation of the age-dependent response. *J Clin Invest* 1993; 91: 465-473.

24. Hamet P., Malo D. and Tremblay J. Increased transcription of a major stress gene in spontaneously hypertensive mice. *Hypertension* 1990; 15: 904-908.

25. Kunes J., Poirier M., Tremblay J. and Hamet P. Expression of hsp70 gene in lymphocytes and hypertensive humans. *Acta Physiol Scand* 1992; 146: 307-311.

Pyrotherapy

The idea of using pyrotherapy to treat certain diseases started with attempts to treat tertiary syphilis (general paralysis) by Wagner-Jauregg in 1918. He induced fever in his patients by injecting infectious agents (malariatherapy). Others followed in his footsteps, and by the 1930s many books and articles had been published on the subject. In the United States, Neymann published a book entitled *Artificial fever produced by physical means* and in France the reference was Richet's book *Pyrothérapie* published in 1935.

This emerging therapeutic technique coincided with a fashion for other physical agents — high frequency currents, x-rays or ultra-violet rays — which attracted certain physicians but aroused the scepticism of others. Naturally this fashion was of interest to physicists and manufacturers. A variety of different machines able to induce artificial fever became available. Hyperthermic boxes, induction coils and electrodes were among the physical methods used to induce hyperthermia. In 1949, Irvine Page published a study of 20 patients with malignant hypertension. With the advent of pharmacotherapy, there have been no further developments in the area of pyrotherapy.

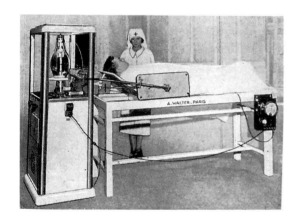 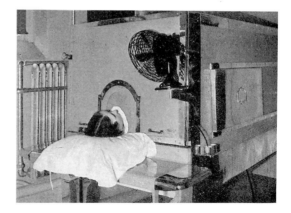

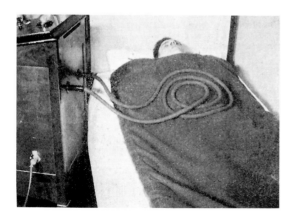 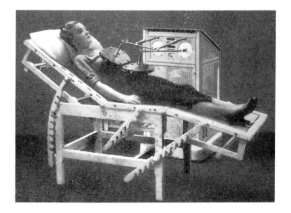

Pyrotherapy: proof of efficacy by examination of the fundus

Just after the second world war, Irvin Page proposed using pyrotherapy to treat patients with malignant hypertension. The results of his trial were published in 1949. Hyperthermia was induced by the injection of Baxter's soluble bacterial pyrogen.

Some patients exhibited marked objective improvement. The photographs below show exudates and haemorrhage in the eyegrounds of a patient with malignant hypertension before treatment (A). After three months of treatment with pyrogen, striking improvement occurred (B).

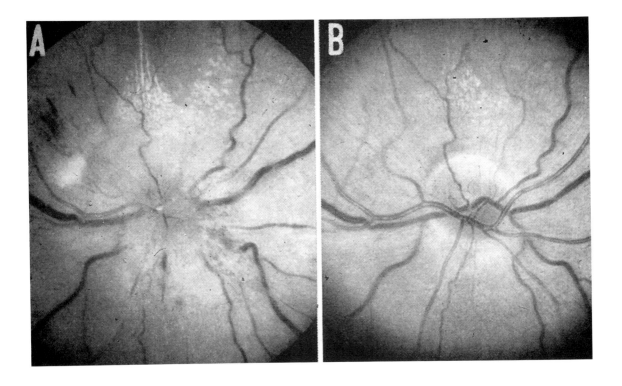

Even polymorphism of one of the HSPs, hep70, was found to segregate with blood pressure [26]. Further studies in this area may reopen new therapeutic interest and improve our understanding of the environment impacting on the expression of hypertension.

SALT FREE DIET AND PROTEIN DIET

Several enlightened authors, such as Huchard, had already indicated the disadvantages of salt for patients with vascular disorders. However it was mainly due to the teachings of Ambard and Beaujard, based on the work of Widal, which marked the true beginning of the salt-free diet. In an important article in 1904 [27], Ambard and Beaujard demonstrated that in patients with Bright's disease, sodium restriction (known as "chloride unloading") was accompanied by a fall in arterial pressure. This was well illustrated in six charts accompanying six case histories. It should be recognised that these authors had no real therapeutic intent and following the example of Achard and Widal, their aim was to emphasise the importance of the relationship between salt load and blood pressure. In their first case, Ambard and Beaujard specified that the reduction in pressure was obtained with ten days of rest and a milk diet. The patient, a 44 year-old man was suffering from cardiac failure (there was no mention yet of asymptomatic hypertension of the type which would be later described by the insurance companies between 1910 to 1920). His arterial pressure, measured with the Potain sphygmo-manometer, fell from 22 to 15 centimetres of mercury at the same time as he excreted 56 grams of salt.

The effect was reversed and the pressure rose again by the administration of the "hospital broth" which contained 10.5 grams of salt per litre. The deduction was that *"there are no other permanently acting hypotensive agents apart from chloride-depleting medication (whence the virtually identical effects of digitalis or theobromine in hypertensive patients, of course without effect in normotensive patients). All other types of medication which act exclusively by direct vasomotor action (nitrites etc), inevitably have a short temporary action. The converse is that no permanent hypertensive agent can exist, apart from medications producing chloride retention (and moreover this ideal medication does not appear to exist). All other medication which acts by vasoconstriction inevitably has a short duration of action (for example adrenaline)"*. This was the beginning of medical control of blood pressure with the treatment of acute clinical situations generally encountered in hospital, and had nothing to do with the concept of risk factors. Initially, the history of antihypertensive treatment and that of cardiovascular or renal therapy were one and the same, namely the treatment of symptomatic patients with renal failure or heart failure who had high blood pressure rather than patients at risk with asymptomatic hypertension. At the time, hypertension discovered fortuitously was not treated.

26. Hamet P., Kong D., Pravenec M., Kunes J., Kren V., Klir P., Sun Y.L. and Tremblay J. Restriction fragment length polymorphism of hsp70 gene, localized in the RT1 complex, is associated with hypertension in spontaneously hypertensive rats. *Hypertension* 19: 611-614, 1992.

27. Ambard and Beaujard. Causes de l'hypertension artérielles (Causes of arterial hypertension). *Archives générales de médecine.* 1904; 1: 520-533.

The salt free diet was not used systematically for populations suffering from hypertension following this publication. This was not, in any case, the authors' intention. They simply maintained that they had *"demonstrated the close relationship between chloride and arterial pressure"*, however they continued to ponder on its pathogenesis: *"Should chloride be seen as the hypertensive agent, or should it only be regarded as an indicator of the retention of suspected, but as yet unproven poisons?"*

During these years, numerous and varied dietary restrictions were proposed for arteriosclerosis, as indeed they were for all diseases. The initial indications of Potain and Huchard, which continued to be recommended by doctors for many years, stressed the importance of the milk diet *"not only because it introduces a minimum number of toxins, but also because it becomes a powerful agent in the elimination of toxins"* [3]. The salt free diet *"is not at all obligatory"*, one still reads in 1913, however it *"is preferable to accustom the patient to restrict the use of sodium chloride, so that should its eventual total removal become necessary, it will be more easily accepted"*, according to a textbook in which hypertension had a whole chapter to itself, in the same way as angina pectoris [28].

On the other side of the Atlantic, the protein theory of hypertension dominated the scene and salt was of less interest. In a lecture given to the American Society for Experimental Pathology in December 1919, Allen expressed his regret about this and praised the ideas of Ambard and Beaujard, *"from the French School"* [29]. Experiments involving small numbers of patients (groups of 2 or 3 subjects) were quoted: in France, as in America, the time of statistical interpretation of therapeutic trials had not yet arrived.

Houghton, in 1922, supported the idea of sodium restriction in hypertension and proposed an intake of less than 2 grams per day [30]. The idea of a salt-free diet in hypertension was making headway. However, those supporting the protein theory still preferred their patients to abstain from a diet too rich in meat. The debate was unresolved. The salt-free diet became popular during the 1940s, encouraged not only by physiopathological considerations, but also because there was a clearer rationale for reducing blood pressure. We should not forget that prior to this period, there were many who still questioned the importance of reducing blood pressure. In 1939, it was still being written that *"there is no dietary treatment which benefits essential hypertension"*. [31]

In the preamble of an important publication [32], Kempner recalled that *"until 1944, the consensus was that dietary treatment was useful in kidney disease, but of no value in hypertensive vascular disease"*. Kempner, who had the financial backing of a life insurance company, undertook

28. Gilbert A., Carnot P. *Médications symptomatiques, circulatoires, hématiques et nerveuses* (Medication to treat symptomatic, circulatory, blood and nervous disorders).1913. Baillière, Paris. p.136.

29. Allen F.M. Arterial Hypertension. *JAMA* March 6th, 1920.

30. Houghton H.A. The treatment of arterial hypertension with low sodium chloride dietary. *Med Rec* 1922; 101: 441-446.

31. Fishberg A.M. *Hypertension and nephritis.* 4th edition. 1939. Lea & Febiger, Philadelphia. Cited by Kempner.

32. Kempner W. Treatment of hypertensive vascular disease with rice diet. *Am J Med* 1948; 4: 545-577.

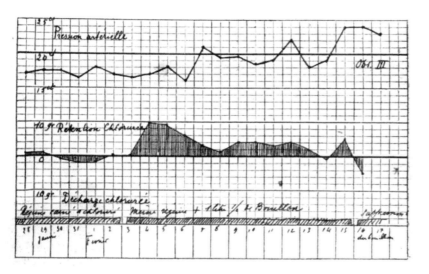

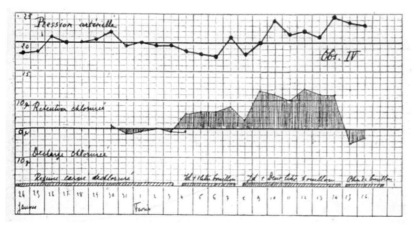

Salt and arterial hypertension: the demonstration of "chloride unloading" from Ambard and Beaujard (1904)

In 1904, Ambard and Beaujard emphasised the importance of the relationship between "*chloride unloading and arterial pressure*" in an article published in the *Archives Générales de Médecine* (charts). Occurring very early in the history of hypertension, this publication had no practical consequences for the diets of hypertensive patients, who, in 1904, were not considered to be suffering from a distinct disease. It was Kempner's work, funded by a life insurance company in 1944, which established the value of the salt free diet.

A PRESCRIPTION FROM 1910: MEDICATION, DIET AND CLYSTER
(according to Huchard)

In cases of arterial hypertension of the "chronic average type":

1. *Take neither tobacco, nor alcohol in any form, nor pure wine, nor liqueurs, nor aperitifs, nor even elixirs or medicinal wine. Never enter an enclosed area where other people are smoking (groups or cafés). Lead a calm lifestyle free from excesses and overwork. Do not become sedentary.*

2. *Diet:*
   At 8 am, have a bowl of milk.
   At midday, eat an ordinary lunch with wine-flavoured water; have neither game, nor fermented food nor food which is high; eat smoked fish and soft cheese.
   At 4 pm, have a bowl of milk.
   At 7pm, have milk soup and a non-meat dish in milk.
   At 11pm, have a bowl of milk.
   To each litre of milk, add one teaspoonful of bicarbonate of soda.

3. *Take one 5g tablespoon of sodium iodide with food, twice daily for 10 days. Drink 300 cubic centilitres of boiled water or take a tablet of lycetol, followed by a glass of Vittel or Evian water.*
   Take one tablet of theobromine 0.5 centigrams, 3 to 6 times daily for the following 10 days.
   Then restart the iodide, and alternate each every ten days.

4. *Every day, perform an intestinal clyster with Esmarch and a long flexible cannula; pass one litre of water which has been recently boiled, containing a spoonful of bicarbonate of soda, into the intestine.*

Commentary. This prescription from 1910 can be judged in retrospect to be ineffective in reducing arterial pressure. It includes ancient remedies (clyster) and at the same time recommends that other age-old medications (the elixir and the medicinal wines) should be abandoned. It is influenced by the medications currently in vogue (iodide and theobromine, which the newly emerging pharmaceutical industry was preparing to use commercially, and the spa waters). The prescription does not forget diet which, in the context of arterial hypertension, reflects the modern approach and highlights the importance of nutritional factors.

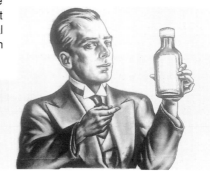

a major investigation which marked a milestone. For a period of four years, 500 patients followed what was called the "Kempner rice diet". Initially, his intention was to demonstrate the importance of a protein diet in hypertension. However he changed his attitude as the facts revealed that with this strict diet, salt restriction itself played a determinant role. Kempner reported that clinically "*a great many patients on the rice diet have experienced relief from headache, dizziness, fatigue, dyspnoea and substernal pain*". As an important rider he stressed that these signs should not be taken as proof of the success of his diet because of their subjective nature. He rightly added that "*only measured results such as decrease in blood pressure, reduction in heart size, loss of edema and reversion of electrocardiogram or eyeground changes should be used to determine the effect of the treatment*". The age of maturity in clinical trials had begun.

SYMPATHECTOMY: THE EFFECTIVENESS OF THE SCALPEL

The first sympathectomy for peripheral arteriopathy was performed by the French surgeon Mathieu Jaboulay around 1900. In 1913, René Leriche demonstrated that division of the sympathetic fibres increased blood flow to the vascular area concerned, due to the arterial vasodilatation produced [33].

Rowntree and Adson took up this idea in 1925 when they performed a bilateral lumbar sympathectomy on a patient suffering from malignant hypertension. [34]. Their idea was to create a diminished zone of resistance in the lower limbs to protect the encephalo-retinal circulation. Following the first trials, it quickly became apparent that the results obtained in the treatment of arterial hypertension by sympathetic denervation depended greatly on the extent of the operation.

The original technique, described and applied by Adson and Craig, consisted of resecting only the splanchnic nerves using a sub-diaphragmatic approach. Bilateral splanchnicectomy using the supra-diaphragmatic approach was clearly more extensive and this was perfected by Peet in 1940 and performed by him on approximately 1500 patients for approximately twelve years [35]. An even more complete sympathetic denervation was achieved by Smithwick's technique, also dating from 1940 [36]. This latter technique combined both the supra and sub-diaphragmatic approaches. It consisted of a bilateral thoraco-lumbar splanchnicectomy performed in two operating sessions, separated by an interval of ten days, using a retropleural, retroperitoneal and transdiaphragmatic approach. The sympathetic chain was resected from the eighth or ninth thoracic vertebra as far as the second lumbar vertebra inclusive and the splanchnic fibres were excised from the middle of the thorax to the coeliac ganglia.

33. Concerning the action of periarterial sympathectomy on the peripheral circulation. Leriche, who was aware of the importance of his approach, published a work in 1933, which is still referred to by historians and philosophers: *Bases de la chirurgie physiologique; essai sur la vie végétative des tissus* (Basis of physiological surgery; an essay on the vegetative life of tissues). 1933. Masson, Paris.

34. Rowntree L.G. Adson A.W. Bilateral lumbar sympathetic neurectomy in the treatment of malignant hypertension. *JAMA* 1925; 85: 959-961.

35. Peet M.M. Results of bilateral supradiaphragmatic splanchni-cectomy for arterial hypertension. *N Engl J Med* 1947; 236: 270-277.

36. The adrenergic mechanisms regulating the circulation of the blood were extensively studied from the beginning of this century and culminated in Alquist's work in 1948 establishing the concept of receptors to explain the diversity of responses to sympathetic simulation. It was well known that arterial pressure elevation was a consequence of the vasopressor and cardioaccelerator effects of sympathetic nerve stimulation or the injection of adrenaline. Moreover, Goldblatt in 1934, had established the renal hormonal theory of hypertension experimentally by demonstrating that ischaemia of one kidney, produced by a clip applied to the artery, caused a lasting elevation of arterial pressure related to the excessive release of a pseudoglobulin, renin, which acted on a substrate of hepatic origin called preangiotonin (angioten-sinogen) to release a vaso-constricting polypeptide, angiotonin (angiotensin) etc. In the minds of certain authors there was a rela-tionship between the sympathetic

This operation, performed by Smithwick on more than 2,500 hypertensive patients over a fifteen year period, was adopted by the majority of teams across the world who used surgery in the treatment of essential hypertension, and sometimes ended in an adrenomedullary curettage.

Prior to the 1960s, the risks of major surgery were justified by the very poor prognosis of patients with severe or malignant hypertension, who within two years of discovery had a mortality rate of 90%. Most of these types of hypertension were already complicated with visceral, encephalo-retinal, cardiac and/or renal alterations. The experience gained in these very unfavourable conditions led the proponents of the method to widen their indications to include young or middle-aged subjects with frank hypertension which was not yet malignant or complicated, with the aim of achieving a significant increase in their life expectancy.

The acceptance criteria for surgery were well documented by Peet, who in his role as neurosurgeon, was sensitive to the clinical and semiological aspects of hypertension [35]. Patients older than 55 were usually excluded, except when they presented with severe hypertensive encephalopathy. Congestive cardiac failure was an absolute indication for exclusion as was severe renal pathology with a blood urea of 1 g/l or greater. Left ventricular failure or a recent history of coronary occlusion represented relative or temporary contraindications only. Effectively, in these conditions, the medium-term prognosis appeared to be too heavily influenced by major irreversible organ failures, particularly with the first two contraindications. For patients who had suffered a cerebrovascular accident, the indication for splanchnicectomy was discussed on a case by case basis, and depended on whether the surgery risked provoking a drop in the cerebral perfusion pressure, particularly orthostatic. Finally toxaemia of pregnancy with persistent hypertension post delivery was considered to be an excellent indication for an extensive sympathectomy, since this involved young women who usually had no major organ failure.

The results of sympathectomy in hypertension were not subjected to scientific analysis as is required today in controlled therapeutic trials. The evaluation of the results must therefore be based on the reports of those who advocated and performed the method.

The mortality from the operation appeared to be low, on average around 2.5% for all groups of mixed degrees of severity [37]. Long-term outcome for the 4 categories of severity, expressed as actuarial survival curves with a mean follow-up of 5 years (maximum 12 years), demonstrated a mortality rate which was always significantly lower among the operated hypertensive patients than among those who had been "treated medically" [38].

and renal hormonal theories of hypertension. Thus M. M. Peet, neurologist and surgeon at Ann Arbor university, thought that hypertension could be caused by the whole process of an exaggerated sympathetic tone affecting the renal vasculature, in turn inducing a bilateral renal ischaemia capable of causing an over-production of renin. (see footnote 35).

37. Smithwick R.H., Thomson J.E. Splanchnicectomy for essential hypertension results in 1,266 cases. *JAMA* 1953; 152: 1501-1504.

38. However, these latter cannot be considered as reliable controls since the group consisted of patients who had refused surgery for various reasons (financial, personal or other) with no correlation as to the severity of their hypertension.

The literature gives little information about the evolution of blood pressure readings in the operated patients. It appears that in the immediate postoperative phase there was a frank reduction, with a tendency for the pressure to increase progressively. In Smithwick's series, 5 years postoperatively, only 45% of patients had a significant reduction in their arterial pressure compared with the preoperative period, while 55% had an unchanged or even higher pressure.

However, the authors emphasised the often spectacular and permanent improvement in severe functional symptoms (headache, dyspnoea, insomnia, problems of cardiac rhythm). This improvement, noted by Peet in 85% of cases, did not appear to correlate clearly with the reduction obtained in the arterial pressure.

Following this pioneering work, sympathetic denervation surgery was widely used by many surgeons, including Smithwick, after whom the operation was named. It was definitively abandoned around 1965. From the mid-1950s, effective and reasonably well-tolerated medical treatment had become available with the diuretics at first, then the centrally-acting drugs such as alpha-methyldopa, and then the betablockers. With these advances in pharmacology, surgical sympathectomy became obsolete.

In the 20th century, medicine has experienced an accelerated pattern of evolution, characterised by continual progress in fundamental knowledge as well as in practical applications. In the treatment of hypertension, extensive sympathectomy marked an important stage, performed as it was over a period of 25 years. One of the merits of this surgical treatment was that it doubtless saved a considerable number of hypertensive patients [39], however it could not address the therapeutic problems associated with a condition as common as hypertension, given the limitations of the method in terms of financial cost and patient suffering. Other areas of medical pathology, such as gastric or duodenal ulceration, also experienced a period of surgical treatment of greater or lesser length, prior to the advent of an appropriate medical strategy.

39. Pickering G. Reversibility of malignant hypertension: Follow-up of three cases. *Lancet* 1971; 1: 413-418.

PENTAQUINE: THE FIRST EFFECTIVE PHARMACOLOGICAL AGENT AGAINST MALIGNANT HYPERTENSION

At the end of the Second World War, there was still no truly effective antihypertensive medication available. In 1946, it was noticed fortuitously during the trial of an antimalarial preparation, (developed by the Squibb Institute for Medical Research) that orthostatic hypotensive episodes were produced in healthy men [40]. The observation of this side-effect raised the possibility that it could be be relevant in the treatment of hypertension. Freis and Wilkins undertook a trial involving 17 patients with moderate or severe hypertension including 3 patients with malignant hypertension [41]. All of the patients were hospitalised for the trial. After

40. Loeb R.F. *JAMA* 1946; 132: 321.

41. Freis E., Wilkins R. Effects of Pentaquine in patients with hypertension. *Proc Soc Exp Biol Med.* 1947; 64: 731-736.

one week, the 3 patients with malignant hypertension noted a reduction in their headaches and cardiac failure, but with no improvement in their renal failure which was already very advanced. For the first time, undeniable hypotensive effects had been obtained with medication. The authors indicated that *"Pentaquine produced a reduction in the vasopressor reflexes, comparable to that obtained by sympathectomy"*. The next question was whether this could rival surgery? Unfortunately, the answer was negative due to severe side-effects and hopes dwindled. The authors of the trial concluded quite candidly that *"toxic reactions to the drug were too frequent and severe to consider its use practicable in the treatment of essential hypertension"*. Although shivering, fever, nausea, vomiting, lumbar pain and lasting hypotension were too great a price to pay for the hypotensive action of the medication, the trial was encouraging. For the first time, malignant hypertension had been improved by medication, and the trial stimulated research into new treatments.

THE ARRIVAL OF THE THIAZIDE DIURETICS:
MODERN PHARMACOLOGY

The diuretics were presented publicly for the first time in Chicago on October 28th, 1957 during the American Heart Congress where Freis presented his results with chlorothiazide [42].

This was a turning point in the history of the medical treatment of hypertension. At last there was an effective oral treatment available, which was better tolerated than the strict salt-free diet and which was capable of potentiating other treatments (allowing a reduction in their doses and therefore in their side-effects).

The January 11th, 1958 issue of the *JAMA* [43] gave a detailed account of the results obtained in 10 patients with chlorothiazide. An 18.7% reduction in pressure, obtained after two or three days, was maintained during the six days of administration of the medication, with the arterial pressure subsequently returning to its initial value. Shortly after the publication of the article, a commentary appeared in the French medical press: *"Chlorothiazide normally produces a a certain degree of diuresis from the first or second day. It can sometimes severely aggravate postural hypotension in cases where this pre-exists. The side-effects are mild and readily reversible on ceasing the medication. The medication potentiates the action of other hypotensive agents; it also increases the hypotensive effect of splanchnicectomy. The mode of action is different from that of other hypotensive agents and it may be secondary to the effects of salt depletion. This medication, which is still under trial, appears to be an interesting new acquisition in the treatment of hypertension"* [44]. The favourable results were confirmed in the *JAMA* of January 10th, 1959 [45].

42. Freis E.D., Wilson I.M., Parrish A.E. Enhancement of antihypertensive activity with chlorothiazide. Presented at the 19th annual meeting of the American Heart Association. Chicago. October 28th, 1957.

43. Freis I. Wanko A., Wilson I., Parrish A. *JAMA* 1958; 166, 133-140.

44. Revue analytique (Analytical review). M. Mouquin. *Arch coeur et vaisseaux* 1958: 505-506.

45. Freis E. Treatment of arterial hypertension with chlorothiazide. *JAMA* 1959. 169; 2: 105-108.

Postoperative changes in the cardiac shadow

Sympathectomy for hypertension was performed for the first time in 1925 and was a notable advance in the care of patients with malignant hypertension whose symptoms could include notably a left ventricular hypertrophy. With advancing knowledge and the prospect of new treatments, the disadvantages of this technique later outweighed the advantages. The last sympathectomies were done around 1965. The study of cardiac volume was an important parameter for evaluating results. The immediate results of a sympathectomy on the cardiac shadow can be observed in an article published in 1955 in *Archives du coeur, des vaisseaux et du sang* and entitled "Extensive sympathectomy in arterial hypertension", R.H. Martin and M. Bonamy.

The first radiograph was taken one month prior to surgery (*figure 1*). The second, taken two months post-sympathectomy, shows the reduction in cardiac volume (*figure 2*) and reveals the presence of clips which mark the extent of the sympathetic ablation: on the right from T2 to L3 and on the left fromT3 to L1.

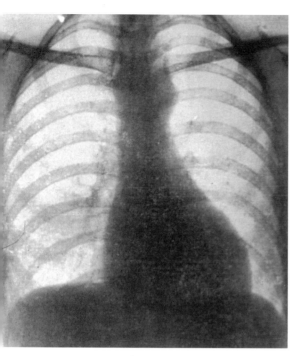

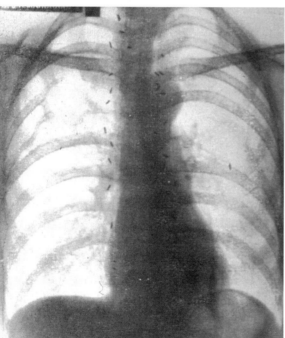

In 1959, hydrochlorothiazide came on the scene. The enthusiasm increased: *"Hydrochlorothiazide exhibits remarkable activity both as an antihypertensive and as a diuretic. The main effect is on the diuresis of sodium and chloride. In 10 patients with arterial hypertension treated with 50 mg of hydrochlorothiazide three times daily, excellent results were obtained in reducing the arterial pressure. The authors recommend that patients enter hospital for the treatment to be supervised, that they receive a sodium-free diet for several days and then receive hydrochlorothiazide and a normal diet"* [46]. At the same time and in the same issue of the *JAMA*, Page and Dunstan published an article on 18 hypertensive subjects treated with guanethidine, with results judged as *"quite favourable"*, but with the appearance of bradycardia and *"rare"* episodes of diarrhoea [47].

The advent of the newer forms of medication did not put an end to the use of older drugs which continued to be widely prescribed. Dosage was modified and it was recognised that when they were used in combination, synergistic activity could reduce the side-effects. In 1958, the combination of reserpine and hydralazine was considered to be the "best medical treatment" for hypertension. The triple combination of reserpine, hydralazine and pentolinium was used in cases of severe hypertension, thus rivalling sympathectomy [48].

Publications on diuretics proliferated and the number of subjects included in clinical trials increased. It was suggested that diuretics should be used in oedema of pregnancy [49]. Owing to their effectiveness, diuretics go down in history as one of the milestones of 20th century therapeutic progress.

The advent of the thiazide diuretics was the fruit of a very effective partnership between chemists, physiologists and clinicians. The therapeutic objective was the development of a medication capable of producing increased sodium and chloride excretion and allowing in the long term, the treatment of pathological states where the expansion of extracellular fluids was thought to play a direct pathogenic (oedema) or indirect (hypertension) role.

The only diuretics available until that time were the mercurials, which had many limitations and contraindications and in practice, there was no valid antihypertensive agent.

It was renal clearance studies in dogs that made possible investigations into the relationship between the structure and activity of several sulphonamide derivatives which led to the selection of chlorothiazide as the first "saluretic" to meet the therapeutic objective. This compound, which has a benzothiadiazine nucleus, proved to be well absorbed by the digestive tract, rapidly active and with an ideal duration of action. It accumulated in the renal tubular cells, where it was secreted into the

46. Mouquin M., Vertes V., Sopher M. Clinical studies on the antihypertensive and metabolic effects of hydrochlorothiazide. *JAMA* 1959; 170: 1272-1273.

47. Page I.H., Dustan H.P. A new, potent antihypertensive drug: Preliminary study of [2-(octahydro-1-azocinyl)-ethyl] guanidine sulfate (guanethidine). *JAMA* 1959; 170: 1265-1271.

48. Orgain, Colin, Munroe, Donnelly. New drugs in the treatment of hypertension. *JAMA* 1958; 166: 2103-2108.

49. Assali, Lewis, Judd, Monds. Clinical and metabolic study of chlorothiazide. *JAMA* 1959; 169: 26-29.

tubular fluid and inhibited the reabsorption of sodium, even when there was metabolic acidosis or alkalosis, a situation in which both the mercurials and acetazolamide became ineffective. Furthermore, chlorothiazide was shown to be well tolerated and its only undesirable effect was its tendency to produce hypokalaemia.

Freis's demonstration of the antihypertensive effectiveness of chlorothiazide in 1957, was a source of gratification for all who had participated in this innovative therapeutic venture. From that time, the thiazides have remained a treatment of choice in hypertension, whether used alone or combined with other classes of antihypertensive compounds discovered since.

THE BETABLOCKERS: "WATERMELON SEEDS, DILUTE HYDROCHLORIC ACID" AND PROPRANOLOL

After the diuretics, the second turning point in the history of the pharmacological treatment of hypertension was the discovery, or rather the commercial availability, of the first specific antagonists of the beta-adrenergic receptors as antianginals first, and later as antihypertensive agents. An important clinical study in 1982 proved their clinical usefulness [50]. Their pharmacological origins go back to 1905, when Langley conjured up the idea of "receptor substances" to explain the observation that sympathetic stimulation (or the administration of adrenaline) simultaneously produced excitatory and inhibitory effects, and postulated that this dual action was related to the respective levels of the two types of receptor substances [51]. The following year, Sir Henry Dale [52] observed that the doses of ergot required to reverse the effects of adrenaline on arterial pressure did not abolish the cardio-accelerator action of the latter. In collaboration with Barger, he expressed the problem in terms of "receptors" and he wrote that *"there has to be something either in the cells, or specifically in contact with them, which has a great affinity for these amines"* [53]. Unfortunately, he rejected Langley's concept for obscure reasons: *"In no circumstances does this mean, as Langley suggests, that there are specific chemical receptors in the cells which are particularly sensitive to these amines"*. Although he was conversant with the work of Clark, Gaddum and Schild (which applied the law of mass action to drug-receptor interactions), he did not adopt the idea of receptors, which because of his high standing in scientific circles, doubtless delayed the acceptance of this theory into medicine. At this stage, people were unaware that some of the amines which were already known, like adrenaline, were actually physiological neurotransmitters.

Between the two world wars, Cannon and Rosenbleuth [54] proposed the idea of transmitter substances, released by the nerve endings and which, following their release, would attach themselves to other

50. Veterans Administration Cooperation Study Group on antihypertensive agents, comparison of propranolol and hydrochlorothiazide for the initial treatment of hypertension. I. Results of short-term titration with emphasis on racial difference in response. *JAMA* 1982; 248: 1996-2003.

51. Langley J.N. On the reaction of cells and of nerve-endings to certain poisons, chiefly as regards the reaction of striated muscles to nicotine and to curare. *J Physiol* 1905; 33: 374-413.

52. Dale H.H. On some physiological actions of ergot. *J Physiol* (London) 1906; 34: 160-206.

53. Barger G., Dale H.H. Chemical structure and sympathomimetic actions of amines. *J Physiol* (London) 1910; 41: 19.

54. Cannon W.B. Rosenbleuth A. Studies on conditions of activity in endocrine organs; Sympathin E and Sympathin I. *Am J Physiol* 1933; 104: 557-574.

substances: the "sympathines". These latter were either excitatory or inhibitory, which explained their dual action. In 1948, Ahlquist established the theory of receptors with its classification of adrenergic receptors into alpha and beta receptors. This conflicted with the dominant view of Dale, Cannon and Rosenbleuth. Ahlquist's views were published by the *American Journal of Physiology* in 1948 in an article which marked a milestone [55].

Ahlquist's discovery was based on the observation that it was the relative strength of action of the sympathomimetic amines which allowed them to be classified into two distinct categories. Adrenaline, followed by noradrenaline, had the most powerful effects. These effects could be both stimulatory (vasoconstriction) and inhibitory (intestinal relaxation) at one category of receptor, which he named alpha. At the other category, which he named beta, isoprenaline (isoproterenol) was the most powerful, followed by adrenaline (epinephrine). Noradrenaline had little or no activity. The beta effects could also be excitatory (cardiac) or inhibitory (extracardiac). Later the sub-classification alpha-1, alpha-2 and beta-1 and beta-2 was accepted.

Moran and Perkins [56] in 1958 observed that dichloro-isoprenaline, a chemical analogue of isoprenaline which had been discovered by Lilly laboratories in a research programme on bronchodilator substances, was able to "block "the stimulant cardiac effects of adrenaline. They therefore suggested that this substance acted on the beta receptors. They re-evaluated the pharmacological effects of phentolamine, phenoxybenzamine and dihydroergotamine and they concluded that these were alpha antagonists. They suggested that the pharmacological agents should be named according to their dominant action, and for the first time they proposed the terms "alpha-blocker" and "beta-blocker".

James W. Black (who since received the Nobel prize and was knighted) established a connection between the pharmacological and clinical aspects and foresaw that the search for products which block the sympathetic cardiac responses would be a clear pharmacological objective. He indicated that experiments had been conducted to evaluate the potential value of these products in coronary disease" [57]. From 1950, Black working at the university of Glasgow had propounded the innovative idea that rather than attempting to increase coronary blood flow to treat coronary disease, it might be more effective to reduce the consumption of oxygen by the heart. In 1959 he was employed by Imperial Chemical Industries to direct a research team working in this field and three years later he proposed using pronethalol [58]. Prenalterol followed next and was produced commercially as an antianginal agent in 1963. This in turn was succeeded by propranolol in 1964.

55. Ahlquist R.P. A study of the adrenotropic receptors. *Am J Physiol* 1948; 153: 586-600. History will record that this article was initially rejected by the editor of the *Journal of Pharmacology and Therapeutics*, because it called into question Cannon and Rosenbleuth's theory on sympathine. This anecdote is of significance because it aptly illustrates how the physiology of this century owed a lot to pharmacology, but also how even at this stage, pharmacologists were loath to admit that they also "practised" physiology.

56. Moran N.C., Perkins M.E. An evaluation of adrenergic blockage of the mammalian heart. *J Pharmcol Exp Ther* 1961; 133: 192-201.

57. Shanks R.G. The discovery of beta-adrenoceptor blocking drugs; in *Discoveries in Pharmacology*, volume 2: "Haemodynamics, Hormones and inflammation". M.J. Parnham and J. Bruinvels Eds., Elsevier Science Publishers BV 1984: 38-72. James W. Black, Project team report, ICI, 1959.

58. Black J.W., Stephenson J.S. Pharmacology of a new adrenergic beta-receptor blocking compound. *Lancet* 1962; 2: 311-314.

It had been observed from the first clinical trials on normotensive subjects suffering from angina, that betablockers caused a significant reduction in arterial pressure [59], so much so, that hypertension was included in the research plan. However it was not until almost 15 years later that the betablockers assumed a place of prominence in the treatment of hypertension, and only then after they had overcome marked resistance to their use in this indication [60]. However, these early times were characterised by indecision, as this retrospective comment from Ahlquist confirms: *"The possible use of propranolol in hypertension has been suggested. Although this has perturbed many people, antihypertensive medications do come and go. I think that you would probably discover somewhere in the medical literature, that almost anything, from watermelon seeds to dilute hydrochloric acid has at one time or another been used successfully to treat hypertension. I hope that propranolol will not fall into this category"* [61].

The more recent history of the betablockers is highlighted by the demonstration of their effect on morbidity and mortality in the treatment of hypertension. The diuretics alone share this demonstration, in the absence of other results from the more recent antihypertensive agents. In the history of the acceptance of betablockers in hypertension, one can also mention Prichard's work on clinical pharmacology [62], the long-term clinical trial of propranolol by Zacharias and colleagues and Hansson's many publications [63].

From a socio-economic standpoint, it is of interest to note the predominance of Anglo-Saxon and Nordic influences, no doubt linked to the large industrial concerns (ICI in Britain and Astra in Sweden). The first large clinical trials were conducted in these countries. It is no surprise, therefore, to find that the largest market for betablockers is also in these countries. It has been more difficult to convince the Latin countries and it has taken longer for the betablockers to be accepted there, but perhaps this is also due to cultural reasons.

ANGIOTENSIN-CONVERTING ENZYME INHIBITORS, OR THE PHARMACOLOGICAL SUCCESS OF THE ENDOCRINE APPROACH

In 1980, the Veterans Administrative Cooperative Study Group contacted various research directors in the pharmaceutical industry to enquire about the possibility of new therapeutic agents. By way of reply, John Alexander, from Squibb, indicated that he needed to undertake a study on a new compound, captopril. He hoped to be able to demonstrate that at low doses this agent would retain its antihypertensive properties without serious side-effects. This study was performed and the results were published in 1982. It opened the way for wide-scale use of the first angiotensin-converting enzyme inhibitor in hypertension.

59. Prichard B.N.C. Beta-adrenergic receptor blockage in hypertension, past, present and future. *Br J Clin Pharmacol* 1978; 5: 379-399.

60. There was a reluctance to use agents which lowered cardiac output and increased peripheral resistance. The discovery of the antirenin properties of betablockers and later the identification of "cardioselective" agents (a better name being beta-1 selective) allowed the betablockers to become key compounds in the arsenal of antihypertensive medication.

61. Ahlquist R.P. Symposium summary, 1967.53. Zacharias F.J., Cowen K.J., Vickers J., Wall B.G. Propranolol in hypertension. A study of long-term therapy 1964-1970. *Am Heart J* 1972; 83: 755-761.

62. Prichard B.N.C. Beta-adrenergic receptor blockage in hypertension, past, present and future. *Br J Clin Pharmacol* 1978; 5: 379-399.

63. Hansson L. The use of propranolol in hypertension: a review. *Post Grad Med J* 1976; 52 (suppl. 4): 77-80.

This pharmacological innovation was the direct end result of knowledge accumulated over 100 years regarding the influence of the renin-angiotensin system in the regulation of arterial pressure.

From the 1940s onwards, several groups of researchers, notably Goldblatt's group, had tried to produce an antirenin serum. The first inhibitor of the renin-angiotensin system which could be used in man was saralasine, discovered in 1971 [64].

The first renin-angiotensin system blocker available was an angiotensin-converting enzyme inhibitor. The history of its discovery began in 1965, the year in which Ferreira isolated a peptide from the venom of a South American snake, the Bothrops jararaca, which potentiated the effects of bradykinin by inhibiting its degradation [65]. At this time, ten years had already passed since the discovery of converting enzyme by Skeggs' team. In 1967, Ng and Vane demonstrated that the conversion of angiotensin I into angiotensin II in the blood is weak or absent in vitro, but is rapid in vivo [66]. As a consequence, the conversion had to occur elsewhere than in the circulating blood (in this case in the lung, where during a single passage angiotensin I is completely broken down into angiotensin II). Ng and Vane completed their experiments with synthetic angiotensin I and, in an article published one year later, noted that bradykinin, like angiotensin I, disappeared completely from the circulation during a single passage through the pulmonary circulation [67]. The product of this degradation possessed a C-terminal end consisting of two proline-phenylalanine amino acids like angiotensin II. They therefore suggested that the same enzyme from the carboxypeptidase family, could be responsible for the degradation of angiotensin I and of bradykinin. In the same year, Bakhle showed that a bradykinin potentiating factor induced the inhibition of converting enzyme [68], and in 1970, Erdös and his coworkers demonstrated that this factor was a dipeptyl-carboxypeptidase [69]. Thus the peptide inhibitors of bradykinin degradation were converting enzyme inhibitors. The way was now open for the invention of a new compound!

Two biochemists from the pharmaceutical industry, Cushman and Ondetti, embarked on this road at the beginning of the 1970s. The administration of a new peptide (teprotide, or SQ 20 881) in man, proved that a converting enzyme inhibitor could almost complete abolish the pressor response caused by exogenous angiotensin I [70]. The clinical effect of this type of treatment was confirmed in hypertensive patients a short time later. Unfortunately, this compound was only active when administered parenterally and Cushman and Ondetti therefore proposed a hypothetical model of the active site of the converting enzyme [71]. In effect, this enzyme possessed numerous properties similar to those of carboxypeptidase A (whose active site had already been described and for which a powerful inhibitor was known). This analogy with

64. This competitive inhibitor of the angiotensin II receptor was basically used as a pharmacological tool, due to its short life and the need to administer it intravenously. Several teams attempted to block renin directly from the end of the 1970s, but were unable to produce a usable agent. Pals D.T., Masucci F.D., Sipos F., Denning G.S. Jr. A specific competitive antagonist of the vascular action of angiotensin II. *Circ Res* 1971; 29:664-672.

65. Ferreira S.H. A bradykinin-potentiating factor (BPF) present in the venom of Bothrops jararaca. *Br J Pharmacol* 1965; 24: 163-169.

66. Ng K.K.F., Vane J.R. Conversion of angiotensin I to angiotensin II. *Nature* 1967; 216: 762-766.

67. Ng K.K.F., Vane J.R. Fate of angiotensin I in the circulation. *Nature* 1968; 218: 144-150.

68. Bakhle Y.S. Conversion of angiotensin I to angiotensin II by cell-free extracts of dog lung. *Nature* 1968; 220: 919-921.

69. Yang H.Y.T., Erdös E.G., Levin Y.A. Dipeptidyl carboxypeptidase that converts angiotensin I and inactivates bradykinin. *Biochem Biophys Acta* 1970; 214: 374-376.

70. Ondetti M.A., Williams N.J., Sabo E. F., Pluscec J., Cleaver E.R., Kocy O. Angiotensin-converting enzyme inhibitors from the venon of Bothrops jararaca: isolation, elucidation of structure and synthesis. *Biochemistry* 1971; 10: 4033-4039.

71. Cushman D.W., Cheung H.S., Sabo E.F., Ondetti M.A. Design of potent competitive inhibitors of angiotensin-converting enzyme. Carboxyalkanoyl and mercapto-alkanoyl amino acids. *Biochemistry* 1977; 16: 5484-5491.

carboxypeptidase A led to the synthesis of a succinyl-aminoacid, SQ 14 225, better known as captopril, discovered in 1977 [72].

THE HISTORICAL BACKGROUND
OF THE CALCIUM ANTAGONISTS

In the mid-1960s, Godfraind and colleagues observed that several substances, including cinnarizine and lidoflazine, at the same concentration prevented the vasoconstriction produced by noradrenaline, angiotensin and vasopressin. These substances also prevented the contractions produced by potassium chloride, which was known to provoke the entry of calcium into contractile cells. The progressive increase in the concentration of calcium in perfusion caused a reversal of the effects of cinnarizine and lidoflazine. The term "calcium antagonist" was coined and used for the first time to describe the properties of the diphenylpiperazines.

In 1963, Knoll laboratories asked Professor Fleckenstein, a physiologist at the University of Freiburg, to analyse the mechanisms of action of verapamil, which up until that time had been considered to be a betablocker [73]. The effects of verapamil on myocardial and vascular tissues resembled those produced by removing calcium from perfusion (and were reversed by the introduction of calcium). Fleckenstein, like Godfraind, concluded from this that this agent interfered with the mediatory effects of calcium on excitation and contraction coupling. As a corollary, the idea of calcium antagonism became an established pharmacodynamic principle. Immediately after the Second World War, chemists at Bayer Laboratories were already busy studying a series of chemical substances derived from the antispasmodic khellin, used in ancient times in the traditional Egyptian pharmacopoeia. Their objective was to find antianginal coronary artery dilators, other than the nitrate derivatives which were the only compounds available at the time, and this led them to the discovery of a new chemical series, the dihydropyridines.The leading compound, Bay a-1040 (nifedipine), was presented to Fleckenstein for assessment of its mode of action. In 1969, he observed that nifedipine possessed the same properties as verapamil, and because of their common mode of action, suggested the existence of a new pharmacological group of substances which he named calcium antagonists.

All of these substances selectively inhibit the flow of calcium ions into the cell. This has been shown by cell physiology studies, particularly those analysing transmembrane ion flow. From a clinical viewpoint, the story of the calcium antagonists began when nifedipine, discovered in 1966 as a powerful coronary dilator, was developed and then produced commercially as an antianginal, first in 1975 in Germany, then in various other countries and eventually, in 1981, in the United States, which was

72. Collier J.G., Robinson B.F., Vane J.R. Reduction of pressor effects of angiotensin I in man by synthetic nonapeptide which inhibits converting enzyme. *Lancet* 1973; 1: 72-74.
Gavras H., Brunner H.R., Laragh J.H., Sealey J.E., Gavras I., Vukovich R.A. An angiotensin converting enzyme inhibitor to identify and treat vasocontrictors and volume factors in hypertensive patients. *N Engl J Med* 1974; 291: 817-821.
Patchett A.A., Harris E., Tristram E.W. et al. A new class of angiotensin-converting enzyme inhibitors. *Nature* 1980; 288: 280-283.

73. Fleckenstein A. History of calcium antagonists. *Cir Res* 1983; 52 (suppl. I): 3-16.

the last country to adopt it due to the stringent FDA regulations. When Attilio Maseri in Pisa and then London, "discovered" spastic angina, the coronary antispasmodic properties of the calcium antagonists produced a great flurry of interest.

From a pharmacological viewpoint, by reason of their chemical and pharmacodynamic diversity, the classification of the calcium antagonists was over-confused. Considering their mode of action compounded this confusion, since the discovery of ion channels of type L and others of type T led to many types of classification being adopted. In an effort to simplify the matter for clinicians, it was proposed to separate diltiazem and verapamil, which were pure calcium antagonists from the dihydropyridines, these latter possessing other actions which added to the inhibitory property on the slow calcium channels [74].

Guazzi and colleagues from Milan were the first to note the antihypertensive effect of nifedipine in coronary and hypertensive patients, but it was the relentless efforts of Fritz Buhler in Zurich during the mid-1980s, which led to the recognition that calcium antagonists had a place in the treatment of hypertension. In particular, Buhler had shown that these agents were of interest in low renin production hypertension, in the elderly and in black patients. The recent concept of vascular selectivity of certain dihydropyridines, the prolonged duration of action of several sustained-release forms of the older calcium antagonists and the availability of long-acting dihydropyridines have allowed these compounds to take a share of the antihypertensive market equivalent to that of the angiotensin-converting enzyme inhibitors and betablockers. However the history of the calcium inhibitors is not one of total success. Hopes for an anti-atherogenic effect have not yet been realised and currently, the results with isradipine in the Midas study have been disappointing.

The dihydropyridines, or at least the first generation ones, have not proved to be of benefit in post-infarct patients and may even have deleterious effects. On the other hand, verapamil is indicated for post-infarct use. Finally, in spite of the methodological imperfections, the retrospective epidemiological work by the Psaty and Furberg group, recently published in the JAMA, casts doubts over the first generation dihydropyridines by revealing that the mortality rate amongst hypertensive patients treated with these compounds is greater than in hypertensive patients treated with betablockers. On the other hand, Pahor's group has shown that verapamil improves the lifespan of hypertensive patients in an equivalent way to the betablockers [75].

74. Materson B.J. Calcium channel blockers. Is it time to split the lump? *Am Hypertens J* 1995; 8: 325-329.

75. Long-term survival and use of antihypertensive medications in older persons. Pahor M.et al. *JAGS* 1995; 43: 1191-1197.

5

THE QUESTION OF NORMS

The fallacy of the dividing line
between the normal and the pathological

"The sublime example was conceived by a physiologist who, having taken a urine sample from a urinal in a railway station where travellers came from all nations, believed himself able to provide an analysis of the average European urine".

Claude Bernard
Introduction à la médecine expérimentale
(Introduction to experimental medicine).
J.B. Baillère, Paris 1865, p. 236

Whereas it is possible to trace the first published accounts of words such as "anaphylaxis", "allergy" or "hormone", the vocabulary of arterial pressure has more obscure origins. The term "hypertension" was not conceived by any single person. Harvey, who discovered the circulation of the blood, spoke in the 17th century of the "force" of the blood, as did Hales and Poiseuille, at the start of the 18th and 19th centuries respectively. Under the influence of experimental medicine this force became "pressure", but the vocabulary used was still directly linked to the current knowledge of physics and hydraulics and it dealt with the mechanics of fluids and not with illness. In the second half of the 19th century, however, the correlation between blood pressure and health was established, with the result that blood pressure was regarded as a system within which variations occurred. Pressure could then be assessed as being too high or too low. Hales had observed that experimental haemorrhage in the mare caused collapse of the blood pressure and ended in the death of the animal. The physical reality of the blood pressure gave rise to the concepts of hyper and hypotension, describing variations occurring outside the "normal" limits, similar to the variations observed in blood sugar levels. But what was the "normal" arterial pressure? This was a banal enough question, but one which must have been asked on a daily basis since the invention of instruments to measure blood pressure and it has certainly stimulated much debate [1].

For yesterday's doctors, as for those of today, it was difficult to define normal pressure and there were numerous obstacles preventing agreement on an unequivocal answer. It was not only physiological variations in arterial pressure which prevented the normal from being described with

[1]. The issues surrounding the normal and the pathological in medicine were brilliantly presented by Georges Canguilhem in 1943. Researchers continue to refer to this work which is a remarkable example of the harmony that can be achieved between philosophical reflection and medical thinking. Anyone wishing to answer the question "what is normal pressure?" would do well to read this book. Georges Canguilhem. *Le normal et le pathologique* (The normal and the pathological). 1943, numerous re-editions by Presses Universitaires de France, Paris.

a single range of figures, but also the various implications inherent in the diagnosis, risk factors and therapeutics which made it impossible for unanimity to be reached. Claude Bernard had defined the normal biological range for blood sugar levels with ease, but blood pressure figures refused to be so easily constrained and there were many problems to be considered, such as the method of measurement, the ages of the subjects, variations in pressure and differences in lifestyles, populations or even the status of the person making the measurement (insurance company doctor, occupational physician, public health doctor, general practitioner, etc.). Thus, there was no single figure for normal arterial pressure, but simply a number of arbitrary "definitions" of normality, which changed as time passed.

FROM CAUSALITY TO A QUANTITATIVE APPROACH

Yesterday's doctor relied on signs and symptoms to define illness. Hippocrates commented at length on his patients' appearance. From this angle, semiology was valuable in defining the character of a disease. Rickets is an example of a descriptive illness. Until the 19th century, it was viewed as a condition of children which caused pigeon chest and twisted legs. Later, as scientific knowledge progressed, the pre-eminence of the clinical definition faded as the advent of endocrinology provided an explanation for the condition which was redefined as a vitamin D deficiency. Likewise, the "fevers", which for centuries were considered as entirely separate illnesses, gave way to purely microbial definitions. Tuberculosis was no longer "consumption and a fever", but a condition caused by Koch's bacillus. From this time on, reasoning in modern medicine was in terms of a scientifically recognised causality [2].

However this evolution in medical thinking, where the importance of the individual was declining in the face of the universality of pathology, could not be applied to hypertension, where there was no "cause" to be discovered. At the beginning of the 20th century, doctors could only make faltering attempts at defining the disease. Certainly it was sometimes possible to explain a raised pressure (particularly in secondary hypertension where an endocrinological or renal origin might apply), but more often such attempts were fruitless [3]. In the vast majority of circumstances, anatomical theories failed to provide an answer and practitioners were forced to abandon their attempts to identify the cause of hypertension, which became "essential" hypertension, a term intended as temporary and criticised from the start, but which is, nonetheless, still used. For lack of anything better, how can essential hypertension be defined other than in terms of numbers ?

In the first half of the 20th century, it was gradually realised that hypertension was an entity that was easier to diagnose and measure than to describe. However this raised a problem, since any reference to a fixed

2. Sinding C. *Le clinicien et le chercheur. Des grandes maladies de carence à la médecine moléculaire* (The clinician and the researcher. From the major deficiency diseases to molecular medicine). 1991. Presses Universitaires de France, Paris.

3. See chapter 3 — Understanding hypertension.

biological landmark refocused attention on the definition of a normal range for blood pressure — a difficult choice with important implications. George Pickering was well aware of this problem and he issued this warning in the opening sentence of an article published in 1955: "*I need hardly stress to you the importance of concepts in medicine. These concepts determine our whole attitude towards the management of the disease and thus, in large measure, the fate of our patients*" [4].

"THE FALLACY OF THE DIVIDING LINE"

Defining a boundary between "normotension" and "hypertension" was necessary for medical practice, but it was an impossible task [5]. When the physician found himself at the patient's bedside, however, he was obliged to interpret the level of blood pressure and decide whether it was normal or pathological. A line between the two, no matter how vague or imprecise, had to be found.

Once the physiologically variable nature of arterial pressure had been recognised and attempts had been made to overcome the numerous barriers to measuring it, clinicians soon turned their attention to defining "normal blood pressure" in man. From 1900 onwards, numerous publications endeavoured to address this problem while others emphasised the arbitrary nature of the boundary between the normal and the pathological [6]. Donzelot, in 1935, spoke of "an approximate value": "*One can accept that hypertension commences at 160 millimeters for the maximum pressure, at 100 millimeters for the mean pressure and at 70 millimeters for the minimum pressure. I must emphasise, however, that these figures represent very approximate values only*" [7]. Allen maintained that " *the normal arterial pressure of the population as a whole is unknown*" [8]. Sir George Pickering alluded to "*the fallacy of the dividing line*" between normotension and hypertension. Reviewing some of the various suggestions in the literature, he stated: "*It is evident that not all can be correct, in fact there is no evidence for any*". He added: "*I have challenged every medical audience that I have addressed in the past 25 years to provide such evidence. The challenge has not been accepted because there is no such evidence*" [9]. A definition for normal blood pressure could not be found.

However not everyone shared this view, since the definition of normotension effectively depended on the goal pursued by the decision-maker. For the life insurance company, the boundary between normotension and hypertension was determined by financial considerations and was located on a risk curve. For the health authorities it was related to questions of public health. In 1939, Robinson noted that it was "*remarkable that the majority of authorities prefer not to define the normal level of arterial pressure, and those that do express their uncertainty by fixing the lower limit for hypertension well below the upper limit for normal pressure, thus leaving a 'no man's land' range of values in between*" [10].

4. Pickering G. The concept of essential hypertension. *Ann Int Med.* 43: 1153-1160, 1955

5. Who would venture to define the minimum height below which a small person is "abnormal"?

6. See chapter 1 — Measuring blood pressure.

7. Donzelot E. *La tension artérielle. L'hypertension, l'hypotension et leur traitement.* (Arterial pressure. Hypertension, hypotension and their treatment). 1935. Baillière, Paris. p. 39.

8. Allen E.V. in Musser J.H. *Internal Medicine 3rd ed.* Lea & Febiger eds, Philadelphia, 1939 quoted by S. Robinson in *Archives of Internal Medicine,* Sept 1939.

9. G. Pickering in: *Hypertension manual. Mechanisms, methods and management.* J.H. Laragh ed. 1973. Yorke Medical Books. N.Y.

10. Robinson S. Range of normal blood pressure. A statistical and clinical study of 11,388 persons. *Arch Int Med*; 64: 409-444, 1939.

For the therapist, the normal level was obscured by the treatment threshold. The number of different approaches which evolved were a function of the state of epidemiological and therapeutic knowledge. The following tables give some idea of the "normal" values quoted in the literature [11].

120/75	Gallavardin (1920)
121/74 (men)	Robinson & Brucer (1939)
124.7 (diastolic pressure not mentioned)	Alvarez (1920)
130/70	Brown (1947)
140/80	Ayman (1934)
140/90	Perera (1948)
140/90	WHO (1959)
150 (diastolic pressure not mentioned)	Cook (1911)
150/90	Thomas (1952)
160 (diastolic pressure not mentioned - women)	Potain (1902)
160 (diastolic pressure not mentioned)	Janeway (1913)
160/100	Bechgaard
170 (diastolic pressure not mentioned - men)	Potain (1902)
180/100	Burgess (1948)
180/110	Evans (1956)

"NORMALITY" AND RISK:
THE LIFE INSURANCE COMPANY EXCLUSION THRESHOLD

During the first 30 years of this century, the insurance companies succeeded in demonstrating that an increase in arterial pressure was accompanied by an increase in mortality [12].

They defined the threshold at which asymptomatic subjects were excluded from cover and described a normal range which was based on financial rather than epidemiological criteria. The Northwestern Mutual Life Insurance Company in the United States adopted the following rule: "*Any subject with a permanent pressure which is 15 mmHg greater than the mean pressure for his age should be rejected*" [13].

These exclusion values were further refined by considering the diastolic pressure. For Gallavardin, the difference between the systolic and diastolic pressure was also important and he observed that there was a proportionately greater increase in the systolic pressure than in the diastolic pressure as hypertension became more severe. In his work he

11. Adapted from Pickering G. See reference 9.

12. See chapter 2 — Recognising hypertension.

13. Quoted by Gallavardin. *La tension artérielle en clinique. Sa mesure, sa valeur semiologique*. 2nd ed. 1920. Masson, Paris. (Arterial pressure in clinical practice. Its measurement and semiological value). The Northwestern Mutual Life Insurance Company gives the following figures. Mean systolic pressures determined following examination of 19,339 subjects: 15 to 20 years, 119 mmHg, 26 to 30 years 123 mmHg, 41 to 45 years, 128 mmHg, 51 to 55 years, 132 mmHg, 56 to 60 years, 134 mmHg. Only 83 out of 2661 subjects aged between 40 to 60 years, who had signed a contract in 1907 and 1910, had died by 1913, which represented just 49% of the mortality anticipated by the current corrected tables. At the same time, data from T. C. Janeway in New York confirmed that elevated systolic pressure had a deleterious effect. His statistics, based on his personal and his father's patients, record the outcome, over a 9-year period, of 458 patients whose systolic pressure was greater than 160 mmHg. During the follow-up, 212 patients died and the cause of death was established in 184 of them. The main causes were renal failure (n = 46), cerebrovascular accidents (n = 29), angina pectoris (n = 10) and pulmonary oedema (n = 7), typical complications of hypertension on target organs. Janeway came to consider any person as hypertensive who repeatedly had a systolic pressure greater than 150 mmHg for young people or 170 mmHg for old people. Janeway T.C. A clinical study of hypertensive cardiovascular disease. *Arch Int Med*. 12: 755-798, 1913.

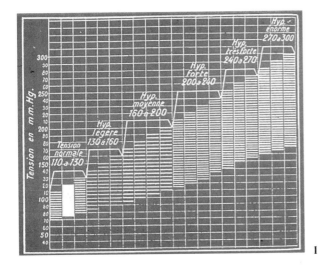

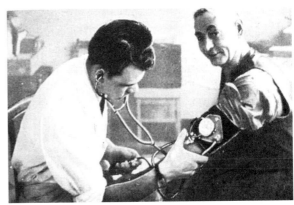

1

2

The arbitary nature of normal pressure: physiological fact, epidemiological mean, risk threshold or treatment threshold?

Very early in the history of pressure measurement, doctors asked themselves where the normal pressure should be placed. At the beginning of the century, Louis Gallavardin proposed adopting a value of 120/75 mmHg. Above this value, he classified pressure as being "mild", "moderate", "severe", "very severe" and "extremely severe" (*figure 1*). Many authors, such as Allen and Pickering, emphasised the arbitrary nature of the diving line between the normal and the pathological, and considered that it was impossible to define this line.

The insurance companies reasoned in terms of risk. The issue here was to define a pressure threshold (often with a systolic of 150 mmHg) above which they would refuse to insure an individual. They soon discovered that the higher the pressure, the greater the risk.

Another approach consisted of adopting as the normal arterial pressure the arithmetical mean of pressures recorded in large population samples. Robinson in 1939 thus proposed a normal pressure of 121/74 mmHg for men and 117/71 mmHg for women.

In 1959, the World Health Organisation recommended that subjects who had an arterial pressure of less than 140/90 mmHg should be considered as "normal" and that those who had a pressure greater than 160/95 mmHg should be considered as hypertensive. With the advent of the first successful treatments for hypertension, the concept of "normal arterial pressure" gradually gave way to the idea of treatment thresholds.

quoted a simple method for verifying whether the differential pressure was normal: the relationship between the systolic and diastolic pressures had to remain approximately constant at around 1.6, as proposed by Josué in 1908. [14].

Where financial goals were involved, normal levels and exclusion thresholds overlapped, and Gallavardin explained this quite clearly: "*If a group of hypertensive subjects is compared with a group of other non-hypertensive individuals, chosen in similar circumstances, it is a certainty that mean survival will be markedly lower in the first group. It is hard to believe that in France, the life insurance companies have not yet developed sufficient concern to insist on blood pressure measurements for their future clients during the medical examination. It is difficult to imagine the sheer number of individuals, obviously seriously affected, whom the companies accept daily on an almost voluntary basis, along with other perfectly healthy individuals who are thus condemned into subsidising the former*" [15].

THE DISTRIBUTION OF ARTERIAL PRESSURE: NORMS AND MEANS

The norm and the mean sometimes had features in common. For the physiologist, the concept of mean pressure was a way of considering the normal [16]. In this context, the normal arterial pressure in man could not be deduced from life insurance statistics based on selected individuals, so that in spite of the insurers' work, Allen wrote in 1938 that "*the norms for arterial pressure in the population at large, as a function of age and sex remain unknown*" [17].

In 1939, Robinson and Brucer published the results of a vast study which included 7,478 men and 3,400 women selected randomly in Chicago and the surrounding area [10]. Here was a large unselected sample which was considered to be representative of the overall population. The arithmetical mean of the arterial pressure was 121/74 mmHg for men and 117/71 mmHg for women. The systolic pressure exceeded 140 mmHg in 10.8% of men and 10% of women. The diastolic was greater than 90 mmHg in 7.3% of the men and in 6.3% of the women. The authors concluded that a definition of norms for arterial pressure based on a population which included both normotensive and hypertensive subjects alike, was questionable. Therefore, for a second statistical assessment, they decided to exclude subjects with an arterial pressure greater than 140/90 mmHg [18]. The results obtained by Robinson and Brucer in this subpopulation demonstrated a mean arterial pressure of 116.3/72.1 mmHg for the men (n = 6854) and 111.6/68.5 mmHg for the women (n = 3015). Their questionable selection of "normotensive" subjects caused a methodological error which was apparent in their study where the effects of age had little influence on the evolution of arterial

14. Josué O. Pression systolique et diastolique. Coefficients cardio-artériels. (Systolic and diastolic pressure. Cardio-arterial coefficients). *Société médicale des hôpitaux*. Feb. 28th, 1908.

15. The linear relationship between the level of pressure and the incidence of cardiovascular complications was still poorly understood. Janeway wrote: "*It appears that no definite prognostic conclusion can be drawn from the height of pressure. This opinion has been confirmed by certain individual cases in which extremely elevated pressure levels were tolerated for six months or more, while other patients with lower pressure levels died within a much shorter space of time...*"

16. See Canguilhem on the concept of the mean (footnote 1).

17. Allen E.V., Musser J.H. *Internal Medicine* 3rd ed. 1939. Lea & Febiger, Philadelphia.

18. This critical level was chosen on the basis of several studies, particularly that of Alvarez and Stanley, who had previously determined the arterial pressure in a large number of subjects. However this study was performed under very special conditions in that measurements had been made on prisoners and their guards. Alvarez W., Stanley L.L. Blood pressure in six thousand prisoners and four hundred prison guards: statistical analysis. *Arch Int. Med* 1930; 46: 17.

pressure, whereas in the population as a whole, pressure increases with age [19]. The arbitrary exclusion of a part of the population led Robinson and Brucer to underestimate the importance of age on the norms of arterial pressure. For them, an arterial pressure of less than 125/80 mmHg was normal. In medicine, however, norm and mean, or rather norm and statistical frequency, cannot be confused.

The problems associated with the definition of the normal arterial pressure were well recognised and discussed by Sir George Pickering [20]. In 1954, his opinion was that essential hypertension does not represent a disease process per se, but that fraction of the population with an arterial pressure higher than an arbitrarily chosen level for reasons that we are unable to explain [21]. This view agreed with the mosaic theory of essential hypertension developed a few years earlier by Page [22]. According to this concept, the variable interaction of several factors can produce an elevation in arterial pressure. This vision of hypertension conflicted with that of Lord Robert Platt, who considered hypertension as a hereditary illness, with a bimodal division of the population into normotensive subjects and hypertensive patients [23].

The concept of hypertension as a quantifiable condition was emerging more clearly. In a study published in 1954, the demarcation between normal and pathological levels was fixed arbitrarily at 150/100 mmHg [21]. However this value represented a working level and was not proposed as an upper limit of normal. The value of 140/90 mmHg proposed in 1948 by Perera, was probably more widely accepted, but there was no true scientific basis for this [24].

In order to facilitate the epidemiological approach, the World Health Organisation in 1959 recommended that subjects who had an arterial pressure of less than 140/90 mmHg should be regarded as normotensive and that those with an arterial pressure greater than 160/95 mmHg should be regarded as hypertensive [25]. Hypertension was said to be "borderline" at levels between 140/90 mmHg and 160/95 mmHg. A statistical study performed in the United States between 1960 and 1962 using the WHO criteria showed that approximately 20% of subjects between 18 and 79 years of aged were hypertensive [26]. The same report also confirmed that arterial pressure increased with age and revealed that prior to the menopause, pressure levels in women were lower than those for men of comparable age, whereas in the older age range, the reverse finding was observed. These data were important because they raised the issue of the definition of normal arterial pressure based on single criteria, without considering the sex, ethnic background or age of the subjects examined.

19. A fact known since 1900-1910.

20. Pickering G. *The nature of essential hypertension*. 1961, Churchill, London.

21. Hamilton M., Pickering G.W., Roberts J.A.F. and Sowry G.S.G. The aetiology of essential hypertension 4. The role of inheritance. *Clin Sci* 1954; 13: 273.

22. Page I. Pathogenesis of arterial hypertension. *JAMA* 1949; 140: 451.

23. Platt R. Heredity in hypertension. *Lancet* 1963; 1:899.

24. Perera G.A. Diagnosis and natural history of hypertensive vascular disease. *Am J Med* 1948; 4: 416-422.

25. World Health Organisation. Hypertension and coronary heart disease: classification and criteria for epidemiological studies. Geneva, *WHO report series* 168, 1959.

26. National Health Survey: Hypertension and hypertensive heart disease in adults. 1960-1962. Washington DC, Department of Health, Education and Welfare, Vital and Health Statistics, series 11, no. 13, US Government Printing Office, 1966.

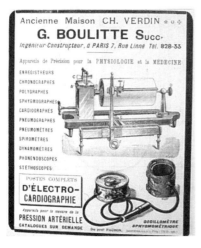

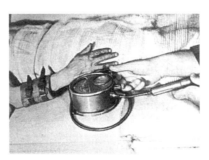

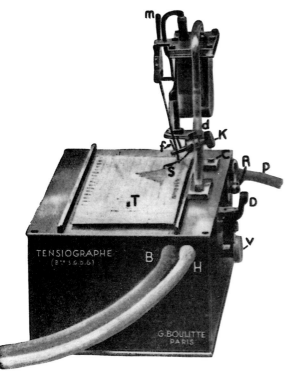

Pressure variations in search of the mean

In the preface of his work "The mean pressure in man in normal and pathological states" (1936), Vaquez indicated that "*it is not our intention to divert doctors from measuring the maximum levels*" but he wanted them to consider more fully "*the infinite number of occasions on which the pressure changes*". In order to measure these variations in arterial pressure, Pachon conceived an oscillograph, which was already on sale in 1912 (top left) and still in use in 1968 (top right). Vaquez judged it to be difficult to use and liable to subjective interpretation and in 1936 suggested a "pressure graph" able to record "oscillographic tracings and which had the advantage of being a permanent record which could be examined at leisure" (bottom).

THE DIAGNOSIS OF ARTERIAL HYPERTENSION BASED ON TREATMENT THRESHOLDS

After the Second World War, the Framingham study demonstrated that cardiovascular risk was directly proportional to both the systolic and diastolic pressure levels. There was a continuous relationship between arterial pressure, myocardial infarction, cerebrovascular accidents and cardiac and renal failure. Hypertension was emerging as a major public health problem. Mass screening and treatment with diuretics and betablockers became the order of the day [27]. With the messages learnt from the large trials, emphasis shifted away from the idea of a normal range of blood pressure towards the notion of treatment thresholds.

The large therapeutic trials performed in hypertension revealed the beneficial effects of treatment on cardiovascular morbidity and mortality. The numerous studies carried out over the years demonstrated that a reduction of 5 to 6 mmHg in the diastolic pressure allowed a reduction in cerebrovascular accidents and myocardial infarction of 42% and 14% respectively [28]. The first therapeutic investigation in 1967 demonstrated that in subjects who had a diastolic pressure greater than or equal to 115 mmHg at the time of inclusion, treatment had a protective effect [29]. Subsequently, patients presenting with lower pressure levels were included. Eventually, the favourable effect of antihypertensive treatment was recognised in subjects whose diastolic pressure was greater than or equal to 90 mmHg [30]. These encouraging results were also noted in older subjects whose elevated pressure had, in the past, been considered to be "normal" [31]. In these patients, the beneficial effect of antihypertensive medication was established in cases of isolated systolic hyper-tension, which was defined as a systolic pressure greater than 160 mmHg associated with a diastolic pressure of less than 90 mmHg [32].

Several countries and international organisations proposed norms for arterial pressure [33]. In all cases, it was recommended that measurements be repeated over a period of several weeks, or even several months, prior to reaching a diagnosis of hypertension. The multitude of approaches confirms that there was still no consensus on the definition of raised arterial pressure, despite considerable efforts in many parts of the world aimed at refining the diagnosis of hypertension [34].

BEYOND THE NORMAL AND THE PATHOLOGICAL DIVIDE: A CULTURAL CHOICE

In medicine the question of what is normal goes far beyond any statistical consideration, because it embraces the ideologies of both the doctor and his patient. For the doctor, anything that interferes with the norm requires him to intervene, while for the subject under examination, it means being designated as a "patient". Thus in everyday practice, statistics trace a boundary between the normal and the pathological

27. See chapter 4 — Treating hypertension.

28. Collins R., Peto R., MacMahon S., et al. Blood pressure, stroke and coronary heart disease, part II: effects of short-term reductions in blood pressure — an overview of the unconfounded randomised drug trials in their epidemiological context. *Lancet* 1990; 335: 827-838.

29. Veterans Administration Cooperative Study Group on Antihypertensive agents. Effects of treatment on morbidity in hypertension: results in patients with diastolic blood pressures averaging 115 through 129 mmHg. *JAMA* 1967; 202: 116-122.

30. Hypertension detection and follow-up program cooperative group. The effect of treatment on mortality in "mild" hypertension: results of the hypertension detection and follow-up program. *N Engl J Med* 1982; 307: 976-980.

31. MacMahon S,. Rogers A. The effects of blood pressure reduction in older patients: an overview of five randomized controlled trials in elderly hypertensives. *Clin Exp Hypertens* 1993; 15: 967-978.

32. SHEP Cooperative Research Group. Prevention of stroke by antihypertensive drug treatment in older persons with isolated systolic hypertension. *JAMA* 1991; 265: 3255-3264.

33. Guidelines of the Sub-Committee of the WHO/ISH Mild Hypertension Committee 1993. Guidelines for the management of mild hypertension: memorandum from a WHO/ISH meeting. *J Hypertension* 1993; 11: 905-918.

34. There is little doubt that in the future consensus will be more difficult to reach with the availability of new methods of measurement, with complex "normal" results. See chapter 1 — Measuring blood pressure.

which separates the two sides. On one side of the divide is the doctor who determines the state of health of the subject under examination, according to the accepted criteria of his time and his scientific culture; on the other side is the individual who no longer decides alone whether he is ill or not. Up until the 18th or 19th centuries, the idea of illness or health depended entirely on how one could cope with one's condition. The normal person was someone whose symptoms did not interfere with his daily needs. In other words, health was a state defined by one's level of tolerance to the restrictions or suffering of one's body. The measurements and newly deciphered physiopathological processes introduced by experimental medicine changed this notion and from then, one could be "in poor health" without experiencing any symptoms. Health, which Leriche elegantly defined in the past as *the progression of life in the silence of the organs*" was losing ground. With experimental medicine, a patient with glycosuria or albuminuria, irrespective of his complaint, lost his state of health and became not ill, but "abnormal".

Claude Bernard asserted that an illness resulted not from any altered state but from a simple distortion of physiology and he reinforced the new status of the abnormal patient who gradually becomes ill by crossing a controversial dividing line. Concerning glycosuria, Claude Bernard indicated that: "*There is no single level of glycaemia, but a condition which is constant and permanent, either within diabetes or outside this state of morbidity. There are only degrees of glycaemia, so that a level lower than 3 to 4 g/l does not produce glycosuria whereas glycosuria occurs above this level. It is impossible to grasp the transition from the normal to the pathological state and there is no more appropriate condition than diabetes to demonstrate the degree of closeness between physiology and pathology*". Elsewhere Claude Bernard stated that "*health and illness are not two essentially different states, as the older physicians believed and some physicians still believe today. In reality, there are only differences of degree. The exaggeration, disproportion and lack of harmony of the normal phenomena constitute ill health*" [35].

35. Quoted by Canguilhem (footnote 1).

The idea that continuity existed in the relationship between the normal and the pathological state began with the arrival of experimental medicine in the middle of the 19th century. In its wake arose a new definition of illness, separated from health by a boundary which was difficult to delineate. The gradual erosion of the symptom which has occurred during the hundred years of hypertension, has played its part in this medical renaissance [36].

36. See chapter 7 — Yesterday's sufferers, today's patients.

Normality is pure fantasy

The concept of "normality" in medicine is an never-ending debate which opposes physicians, scientists and philosophers. The definition of "normal" blood pressure depends to a large extent on the examiner and his objectives: insurance agent, statistician or therapist. An article published by G.W. Pickering in the Annals of Internal Medicine in1955 (43;1153-1160) made a considerable impact on this debate. Three short extracts are reproduced below.

"I need hardly stress to you the importance of concepts in medicine. These concepts determine our whole attitude to the management of the disease and thus, in large measure, the fate of our patients".

"My first point is that the practice of making a sharp division between normal and pathologically high pressure is entirely arbitrary and is in the nature of an artefact. Essential hypertension represents the upper end of a distribution curve showing continuous variation, with no definite evidence of two populations".

"All these arguments thus suggest that there is no justification for a division of arterial pressures into normal and pathologically high, and that it is the height of the pressure that matters. In fact, arterial pressure seems to behave as a graded characteristic: the differences between the lower pressure and the higher are quantitative, not qualitative; they are differences of degree, not of kind".

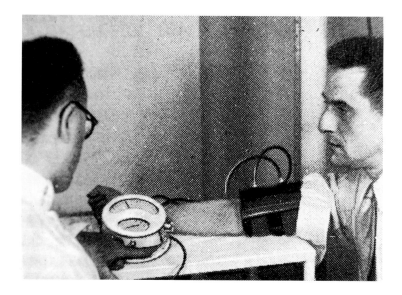

6
SOCIAL PRESSURES

Migration and nutrition: hypertension divided between genetics and the environment

"The more one thinks about it, the more one realises that this [primitive] state was the most secure and the best suited to man. If he was compelled to abandon it, it must surely have been through some tragic twist of fate which, for the common good, ought never to have occurred. The example of savages that we have found living in this state would tend to confirm that the human race was created to remain so forever, for this is the true youth of our world. Each subsequent advance has been a step towards the imperfection of the individual and the decrepitude of the species".

Jean-Jacques Rousseau
Discours sur l'inégalité
(Discourse on inequality)
1775

Good health is dependent on the environment. The ancient Greek physicians were well aware of this and an entire volume of the Hippocratic collection was devoted to this subject [1]. As early as 500 BC, the interrelationships between health and the environment were being studied [2]. It is beyond the scope of this work to summarise these 25 centuries of medicine. Before the era of blood pressure measurement, hygienists (who were not yet called epidemiologists) were already studying the influence of alcohol, diet and the emotions, and they strongly suspected that these factors could increase the incidence of apoplexy, angina or arteriosclerotic degeneration of the blood vessels [3]. The emergence of hypertension as a clinical entity in the early 20th century did not introduce any fundamentally new element into this debate. Physicians studying hypertension adapted the approach to the ever-evolving circumstances of modern life. By looking at such factors as alcohol, geographical location, urban life and salt content of the diet, they were simply climbing on the environmental bandwagon. They went even further and, during the colonial period, extended their studies to distant lands travelling the world to measure blood pressure in "native populations living in the Tropics" [4].

There is a dual interaction between blood pressure and medico-social factors. On the one hand, there are social and cultural factors which tend to increase blood pressure levels in the population as a whole,

1. It is entitled *Air, water and places.*

2. Some people are of the opinion that this Hippocratic approach was a key element in the founding of the human sciences. Jouanna J. *Hippocrates.* 1992. Fayard, Paris.

3. The effect of tobacco was hardly studied, if at all.

4. Margrave and Sison. Blood pressure in the Tropics. *The Philippine Journal of Sciences* 1910; 5: 325.

and on the other hand, there is "medical activity" in the broad sense which, particularly since 1970, has devoted considerable energy and expense to lowering the blood pressure of individuals considered to be "hypertensive". The description and discussion of these interractions have given rise to an abundance of articles in the medical literature which will be briefly reviewed later, but a preliminary remark is in order. A "sociological" approach to hypertension cannot be reduced to a simple epidemiological analysis — statistics do not explain everything. Thus, the statistics produced by the insurance companies, for all their worth and innovativeness, which we emphasised in a previous chapter, were sometimes misleading. In the not so distant past, insurance company physicians wrote a lot of nonsense about the longevity of races [5]. With this in mind, we must humbly recognise that some of the modern views on the influence of social, cultural and racial factors on hypertension may not stand the test of time. One must not forget that after all, blood pressure is not a sociological parameter but a physiological one.

BLOOD PRESSURE ELEVATIONS DIVIDED BETWEEN THE "INNATE" AND THE "ACQUIRED"

Hypertension does not affect all populations and individuals in the same way. Certain ethnic groups and social categories are harder hit than others. These differences have been particularly well studied in the United States where the black population has a higher prevalence of hypertension [6]. The mortality associated with hypertension follows the same pattern so that the rich and the poor are not equal in the face of cardiovascular risk. Numerous factors associated with "social pressure" such as alcoholism, unemployment, insecurity and stress, increase the incidence and severity of hypertension [7]. The environment has a strong influence on the general health of a population, including its blood pressure levels. But the recordings made by our manometers are subject to interpretation errors and must be viewed with circumspection. While statistics on such things as occupational accidents provide reliable and easily quantifiable medico-social information, the mean blood pressure of a group cannot be considered in the same light. Having said that, there are a number of well-identified dietary, social and psychological factors which are clearly associated with blood pressure. There is, however, an additional difficulty and that is that hypertension also depends on genetic factors which are not subject to the same laws as sociology, nutrition or "stress". Any discussion on social pressures must necessarily take into consideration the respective contributions of the "innate" and the "acquired" [8]. A complex issue indeed !

Notwithstanding the genetic contribution to blood pressure control, it has emerged from all the epidemiological enquiries performed that hypertension cannot be dissociated from social factors. We are obliged

5. Stévenin H. *La Médecine d'assurance sur la vie. Facteurs biologiques, médicaux et sociaux de la mortalité et de la longévité* (Life insurance medicine. Biological, medical and social factors of mortality and longevity). 1951. Masson, Paris.

6. According to the NHANES III study, the age-adjusted prevalence is 32.4% for black Americans, 23.3% for non-Hispanic white Americans and 22.6% for Hispanic Americans. Kaplan N.M. *Clinical hypertension* Sixth ed. 1994. Williams & Wilkins, Baltimore.

7. It is interesting to note that medical inequalities dependent on social factors were documented and denounced as far back as the 18th century. 200 years later, in a totally different epidemiological context, the progress in medical care has had little effect on the sociological component of an individual's state of health.

8. Studies on the prevalence of hypertension in certain families or ethnic groups suggest that predisposition may be present at birth (see chapter 8 on the genetics of hypertension). But in addition to purely genetic factors, the "innate" may also refer to non-hereditary prenatal events. Several studies have drawn attention to the relationship between birth weight and blood pressure in adulthood, the risk of hypertension being particularly high if birth weight is low compared to placental weight. Genser G., Rymak P., Isberg P.E. Low birth weight and risk of high blood pressure in adulthood. *Brit Med J* 1988; 296: 1498-1500.

to recognise that the "chemical fault" (i.e. the gene or secondary hypertension resulting from an identifiable endocrine abnormality) sometimes responsible for hypertension is less prevalent in the millions of people with essential hypertension than what we might call the "social fault". The theory according to which hypertension results from a lifestyle that is poorly adapted to an individual's genetic make-up tends to reconcile these two views. This is what we suggest in the section to follow — with all its uncertainties.

BECOMING HYPERTENSIVE : THE REMARKABLE EXAMPLE OF MIGRATING POPULATIONS

Broadly speaking, there is a tendency for migrating populations to acquire the diseases of their adopted homelands. Hypertension is no exception to this rule. Populations living outside the industrial world often suffer little from hypertension. In these populations, blood pressure does not increase with age — they are referred to as "low-blood pressure populations". Such populations have been documented in many different parts of the world. They include the Eskimos, the Australian aborigines, the nomad tribes of Kenya, Pygmies in the Congo, Melanesian and Polynesian tribes or the Indians of South America. Remarkably, these populations usually become hypertensive when they migrate to industrialised areas [9]. This phenomenon has been reported in cross-sectional studies, which have been open to criticism, but the data have been confirmed in prospective longitudinal studies.

For example, the inhabitants of the Tokelau islands who emigrated to New Zealand had a rise in their blood pressure which paralleled the increase of sodium intake [10]. Similar observations have been made in members of a so-called "low pressure" Kenyan tribe migrating to an industrialised area [11]. Likewise increasing blood pressure levels were observed in Ethiopians migrating to Israel. The incidence of hypertension in this population increased three-fold and they also acquired other risk factors such as hypercholesterolaemia and hyperinsulinism [12].

A recent study looked at young Somalis immigrating to Italy. In the first six months following their arrival, they exhibited a significant increase in both systolic and diastolic blood pressure evaluated by 24-hour blood pressure monitoring [13]. Simultaneously, 24-hour urinary sodium excretion increased and plasma renin activity decreased. The increase in blood pressure was correlated with that of urinary sodium excretion. These observations should not, however, conceal the fact that certain populations have conserved a remarkably low incidence of hypertension despite an increasing incidence of obesity and insulin resistance. This situation probably reflects a predominant genetic influence.

9. Where their blood pressure levels often exceed those observed in the indigenous population.

10. Beaflehole R., Salmond C.E., Hooper A. et al. Blood pressure and social interaction in Tokelauan migrants in New Zealand. *J Chron Dis* 1977; 30: 803-812.

11. The rise in blood pressure paralleled an increase in body weight and consumption of alcohol and sodium. Poulter N., Khaw K.T., Hopwood B.E.C. et al. Salt and blood pressure changes due to urbanization. A longitudinal study. *J Hypertens* 1985; 3 (suppl 3): 375-377.

12. Goldbourt U., Khoury M., Landau E. et al. Blood pressure in Ethiopian immigrants: relationship to age and anthropometric factors, and changes during their first year in Israel. *Isr J Med Sci* 1991; 27: 264-267. Bursztyn M., Rar I. Prediction of hypertension by the insulinogenic index in young Ethiopian immigrants. *J Hypertens* 1995; 13: 57-61.

13. Modesti P.A., Tamburini C., Hagi M.I., Cecioni I., Migliorini A., Serneri G.G.N. Twenty-four-hour blood pressure changes in young Somalian blacks after migration to Italy. *Am J Hypertens* 1995; 8: 201-205.

HYPERTENSION IN BLACKS: A QUESTIONABLE ENTITY

The black population of the United States is an important example of a transplanted group whose blood pressure is higher than that of subjects remaining in their original homeland (sub-Saharan Africa) and that of the population of their adopted homeland. This difference has been attributed to general causes such as "psycho-social stress" and the plight of an underprivileged minority. Black Americans have higher sodium retention than Whites and therefore exhibit a greater increase of blood pressure than the latter for an equivalent sodium load. They also have lower renin levels which might reflect this tendency to conserve an excessive amount of sodium. This trait, probably of genetic origin, is an obvious advantage in terms of survival for populations who live in a tropical climate and who have limited access to sodium. In contrast, it might be a disadvantage for populations who live in temperate climates and who have free access to sodium which is a source of expansion of extracellular fluid and hypertension.

In an attempt to explain certain characteristics of sodium regulation, Blackburn and Prineas have put forward an interesting hypothesis called the "slave" hypothesis [14]. Black Americans, originally from Africa, were transferred to the American continent during the slave trade. They travelled under appalling conditions of hygiene where malnutrition, diarrhoea and vomiting took an extremely heavy toll. Blackburn and Prineas suggest the hypothesis that subjects who best retained sodium, for genetic reasons, were probably the ones who best survived this terrible ordeal. According to the hypothesis, this resulted in a sort of genetic selection whereby the individuals who arrived in the New World were those who best retained sodium. If this is true, it would be logical to observe a particular high incidence of hypertension in their descendants [15].

It should be pointed out however that this theory has been widely challenged. In particular, the increased pressor response of Blacks to acute or chronic variations in salt intake is by no means specific of Blacks living in the United States. The higher incidence of hypertension in Blacks in the United States (and in Europe as well) has led to the individualisation of "hypertension in black populations". The controversy over this "entity" is interesting for two reasons. Not only does it raise the problem of the innate and the acquired in hypertension, but it also highlights the methodological problems of epidemiology.

The special features of this form of hypertension (frequency of complications, low renin and sensitivity to diuretics) are well known to clinicians and do indeed appear to support the idea of a homogenous group. Specific responses to various classes of antihypertensive drugs have been demonstrated in a number of studies. In contrast, the opponents of a specific form of hypertension in Blacks put forward two types of arguments. The first is that blood pressure levels are very different in

14. Blackburn H., Prineas R. Diet and hypertension: anthropology, epidemiology, and public health implications. *Prog Biochem Pharmacol* 1983; 14: 31-79.

15. Wilson T.W., Grim C.E. Biohistory of slavery and BP differences in Blacks today. *Hypertension* 1991; 17 (suppl. 1): 122-128.
Wilson T.W., Hollifield L.R., Grim C.E. Systolic BP levels in black populations in sub-Saharan Africa, the West Indies, and the United States: a meta-analysis. *Hypertension* 1991; 18 (suppl. 1): 87-91.

Blacks living in the United States and those remaining in their African countries of origin. Certain ethnic groups in Africa even have a markedly low level of blood pressure. The second argument, which is a corollary of the first, is that environmental factors can almost always be demonstrated to explain the differences in blood pressure [16]. In fact, the concept of "black subjects" is not simply a question of skin colour, and factors such as history, culture and socio-economic status etc. cannot be neglected. The closer one looks at these factors, the clearer it becomes that there is no statistical correlation between blood pressure level and skin colour. Futhermore, the gene for sickle cell disease, considered to be a typically "black" disorder, has been correlated with a low level of blood pressure [16]. In summary, hypertension in black subjects is the best example of a population in which the prevalence of a disease is low in the country of origin, high in the country of adoption and for which it is impossible, despite a considerable mass of work, to separate out the genetic and environmental factors.

WEIGHT, ALCOHOL AND SODIUM:
A SOCIETY OF OVERABUNDANCE

The association between obesity, diabetes and hypertension is now well established. In fact, obesity has never been well regarded in medicine and even at the end of the 19th century, individuals who were overweight were suspected of being likely candidates for apoplexy. As early as 1914, insurance companies demonstrated the existence of a correlation between life expectancy and abdominal circumference. The statistics from other companies corroborated these results, in particular the Medical Impairment Study (1929), which looked closely at this aspect [17]. It was during the same period that the relationship between blood pressure and obesity was first noted, which indicates how striking this relationship is [18].

Hypertension is 3 to 6 times more frequent in obese individuals than in non-obese subjects [19]. Before the age of 30, it has even been reported that the risk is increased 30-fold. The Intersalt Study revealed a strong and independent correlation between body weight and blood pressure, both systolic and diastolic. A causal relationship is substantiated by the drop in blood pressure which accompanies weight loss.

It is interesting to note that in Fabre's study on staff members of an international organisation, the prevalence of obesity in an ethnic group does not necessarily correlate with that of hypertension [20]. However, this discrepancy does not show up in all studies.

The correlation between obesity and blood pressure is also present in the "syndrome X" which associates hypertension, obesity and diabetes, three conditions which are closely interrelated from an

16. Lang T. L'entité hypertension artérielle du "sujet noir" (Hypertension in Blacks). *Presse méd* 1994; 23:1642-1645.
Rostand S.G. Hypertension et insuffisance rénale chez les Noirs: rôle des facteurs génétiques et des facteurs liés à l'environement (Hypertension and renal failure in Blacks: the role of genetic and environmental factors). *Actual Néphrol Hôp Necker.* 1991. Flammarion Médecine-Sciences, Paris. pp. 117-132.

17. Cited by Stévenin H. in: *La médecine d'assurance sur la vie* (Life insurance medicine). *op cit.*

18. Coburn. Substandard Life Insurance. Trans For Act 1929.

19. Cambien F. Relation entre l'excès de poids et l'hypertension artérielle (Relationship between excess body weight and arterial hypertension). *Nouvelle Presse Méd* 1982; 11: 3641-3645.
Kannel W.B. Brand N., Skinner J.J. The relation of adiposity, blood pressure and development of hypertension: the Framingham study. *Ann Int Med* 1967; 67: 48-56.

20. Fabre studied blood pressure levels in staff members of an international organisation. The subjects came from many different countries, all lived in Geneva, lunched at the same cafeteria, had the same employer and had all more or less adopted a "western" lifestyle. Although not all the environmental factors had been accounted for (in particular urinary sodium excretion was not measured), the differences in blood pressure between ethnic groups was clearly more striking than their differences in lifestyle. Fabre J., Backzo A., Laravoire P., Dayer P., Fox H. Hypertension artérielle et facteurs ethniques (Arterial hypertension and ethnic factors). *Actual Néphrol Hôp Necker.* 1982. Flammarion Médecine-sciences, Paris. pp. 27-42.

epidemiological standpoint. The incidence of hypertension is markedly increased in obese patients and insulin-dependent diabetics. In contrast, many subjects with essential hypertension exhibit abnormal glucose tolerance and hyperinsulinism, even in the absence of obesity. Various studies in large populations have shown that there is a correlation between plasma insulin and blood pressure. Plasma insulin also correlates with triglyceride levels and with an android pattern of body fat distribution (evaluated by the waist/hip ratio). This resistance to insulin has been confirmed in various series of obese or non-obese hypertensive subjects by the "insulin clamp" technique. It has been suggested that insulin resistance with hyperinsulinism might be the common denominator for diabetes, obesity and hypertension [21].

It has even been stated that hypertension is a metabolic and not a vascular disease. This concept, individualised by Reaven [22] under the name "syndrome X" has attained a level of popularity which probably exceeds what the facts actually show. Nevertheless, it does draw attention to an essential link between obesity, diabetes and hypertension.

BLOOD PRESSURE AND ALCOHOL:
OLD WINE IN NEW BATTLES

The condemnation of the dangers of excessive alcohol intake far preceded the measurement of blood pressure. From the middle of the 19th century, hygienists and physicians medicalised this condemnation and invented the word "alcoholism". From then on, excessive alcohol consumption was no longer simply a source of family ruin or a cause of police intervention for unruly behaviour, it had attained the status of a disease [23] responsible for liver cirrhosis, epilepsy, madness, and more generally the corruption of the race.

In his superb Dictionary of preconceived ideas (Dictionnaire des idées reçues), Gustave Flaubert (quite a drinker himself) gave this definition: "*Alcohol: the cause of all diseases*". The invention of the sphygmomanometer did not contradict him: "*Alcohol is the cause of hypertension*" declared Camille Lian in 1915 before the Academy of Medicine. Serving as an army physician at the time, Lian used the Pachon-Lian sphygmomanometer to measure the blood pressure of 150 subjects divided into 4 groups: "sober, average drinkers, heavy drinkers and very heavy drinkers". The results were revealing: 25% of "very heavy drinkers" and 17.5% of "heavy drinkers" had a blood pressure "clearly" exceeding 150/100 [24].

Chronic alcohol intake raises blood pressure independently of body weight. Hypertension is 2 to 3 times more common in chronic drinkers than in non-drinkers. The Framingham study showed a J curve: blood pressure is slightly higher in non-drinkers than in occasional drinkers.

21. Ferrannini E.et al. Insulin resistance in essential hypertension. *New Engl J Med* 1987; 317, 350-357.

22. Reaven G.M. Role of insulin resistance in human disease. *Diabetes* 1988; 37, 1595-1607.

23. Didier Nourrisson. *Le Buveur du XIXe siècle* (The 19th century drinker). 1990, Albin Michel, Paris.

24. Lian C. L'alcoolisme, cause d'hypertension artérielle (Alcoholism, cause of arterial hypertension). *Bull Acad méd* 1915; 74: 525-528.

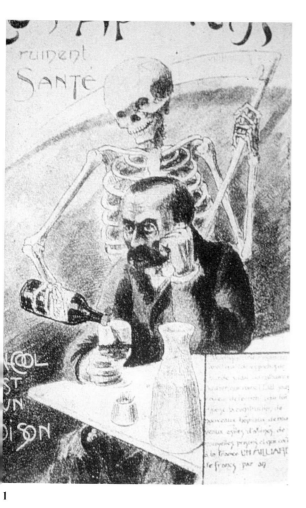

1

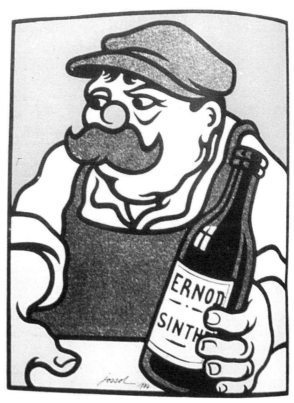

2

Alcoholism, a cause of hypertension

In 1915, Camille Lian, in a communication to the Academy of Medicine, demonstrated quite remarkably that "*alcoholism is a cause of arterial hypertension*". By recording daily wine consumption (in litres and not in glasses as today) in 150 military personnel aged 42 or 43, he noted that in the group of "very heavy drinkers" (i.e. 3 litres of wine per day and more) 25% were hypertensive while amongst "heavy drinkers" (2 to 2.5 litres of wine per day) the prevalence was 17.5%. He remarked that their blood pressure was well above the normal defined as 150/100 mmHg measured with the Pachon-Lian sphygmomanometer. In the early part of the 20th century, anti-drinking leagues published postcards, posters and leaflets designed to terrify the consumer (*figure 1*). Concomitantly, advertising became a formidable means of encouraging consumption (*figure 2*).

In contrast, beyond a certain threshold, the increase in alcohol consumption was accompanied by a proportional increase in blood pressure. In the Intersalt study, there was a significant correlation between blood pressure and alcohol intake in 35 of the participating centres and there was also a between-centre relationship [25].

There is a causal relationship between blood pressure and alcohol and several studies have shown that by reducing the consumption of alcohol, blood pressure can be lowered. In addition, alcohol appears to have a very negative influence on compliance with antihypertensive therapy.

SODIUM AND OTHER CATIONS

The relationship between sodium and hypertension is considered to be one of the most crucial between an environmental factor and the level of blood pressure [26]. Population studies have shown that the prevalence of hypertension increases as sodium consumption increases and rather audacious mathematical transformations have established a positive quantitative correlation between sodium consumption and the level of blood pressure or the prevalence of hypertension [27]. By means of more classical methodology, the Intersalt study came to the same conclusion but expressed it in conspicuously more cautious terms [28]. The fact remains that populations who consume little salt definitely have a low incidence of hypertension and those with a high salt consumption have a much higher incidence. The spectacular difference in blood pressure between Japanese living in the north and those living in the south is a classic example.

However, the correlation between salt consumption and blood pressure becomes less obvious at the level of the individual unless extravagant mathematical artefacts are used [29]. In the Intersalt study, within-centre correlations between urinary salt excretion and blood pressure disappeared if the results were adjusted for body weight and alcohol consumption.

Differences in salt intake represent an important factor underlying the differences in blood pressure between populations, and yet this factor is difficult to demonstrate between individuals of the same population. This no doubt reflects another facet of the genetics-environment dichotomy. The concept of blood pressure sensitivity to sodium has inspired numerous studies. It is probably a key factor and very likely genetically determined [30]. It appears that sensitive subjects have a relative expansion in extracellular fluid and a low renin level which cannot be readily stimulated.

The real question is probably not whether sodium is responsible for hypertension or not, but rather whether a given individual has salt-sensitive hypertension. It is an inescapable fact that salt balance (dependent on kidney function alone) and hypertension are intimately linked.

25. Many other studies in Australia, Germany and other countries have confirmed this relationship. Lang et al., in a cohort of 6,665 subjects in France showed that there was a very significant correlation between alcohol consumption and blood pressure. The prevalence of hypertension for men and women combined was 24.3% in subjects who consumed more than 6 glasses of an alcoholic drink daily versus 11.3% in non-drinkers. Lang T., Degoulet P., Aime F. et al. Relationship between alcohol consumption and control in a French population. *J Chron Dis* 1995; 40:713-720.

26. The vital importance of salt, not only physiologically but also culturally, regiously and economically, has inspired numerous historical, anthropological or medical treatises on the subject.

27. Law M.R., Frost C.D., Wald N.J. By how much does dietary salt reduction lower blood pressure? I) Analysis of observational data among populations. *Brit Med J* 1991; 302, 811-815.

28. Intersalt Cooperative Research Group. An international study of electrolyte excretion and blood pressure. Results for 24 hour urinary sodium and potassium excretion. *Brit Med J* 1989; 297, 319-328.

29. Frost C.D., Law M.R., Wald N.J. By how much does dietary salt reduction lower blood pressure ? II) Analysis of observational data within populations. *Brit Med J* 1991; 302: 815-818.

30. Muntzel M., Drüeke T. A comprehensive review of the salt and blood pressure relationship. *Am J Hypertens* 1992; 5: 1S-42S.

Convincing proof of this relationship has been provided by renal transplant studies in animals and even in man [31]. The bottom line is that genetically salt-sensitive individuals become hypertensive if they consume too much salt, and managing this type of hypertension involves modifiying salt balance through diet or drugs (diuretics).

Many other nutritional factors have been accused of influencing the blood pressure of populations but alcohol, salt and obesity are by far the most important ones. The role of dietary potassium and calcium are hotly debated but they do not easily lend themselves to a "sociological" analysis. Unlike salt, alcohol and obesity, calcium and potassium consumption are less dependent on cultural or social factors.

HYPOTHESIS: HIGH BLOOD PRESSURE REFLECTS THE INCOMPATIBILITY BETWEEN LIFESTYLE AND GENETIC MAKE-UP

The influence of the environment on a pre-determined genetic make-up has not escaped the attention of anthropologists. Eaton [32] considered that genetically speaking, human beings today were still the hunter-gatherers of the stone age transported by time into a world which differs radically from that for which our genetic constitution was selected. The human genome has not changed very much in 10,000 years, but during that same period, our culture has been transformed to such an extent that there is now an incompatibility between our old, genetically determined biology and certain essential aspects of our daily lives. The result is a number of "diseases of civilisation" which are the cause of 75% of all deaths in Western nations but which are rare in populations whose lifestyle has remained similar to that of our pre-agricultural ancestors. Eaton compared the diet of average modern Americans with what one can postulate to be the diet of their hunter-gatherer ancestors (based on the diet of the most primitive pre-agricultural communities still in existence today). Eaton estimates that our ancestors had a diet which was lower in fat, and based on polyunsaturated fats, consumed less sodium, more potassium and more fibre. According to this view, hypertension is a disease of cultural adaptation, the inevitable consequence of a lifestyle increasingly unadapted to our genetic make-up. The main factors are overeating and a diet too rich in salt and saturated fat, combined with alcohol and more recent "defects" of so-called modern society.

This way of looking at things has given rise to simplistic clichés which have more to do with ideological trends than with scientific fact. Medical treatises of the 19th century are full of such stereotypes. For example, yesterday's celebrated gout sufferer, portrayed as a podgy, jovial, well-fed and well-inbibed individual, is no longer seen in the same light. Today he is viewed as a likely candidate for an early and well-deserved death, and not simply as the victim of a chronic disease [33].

31. The nature of this congenital abnormality of the urinary sodium/blood pressure relationship is not well understood. Amongst the possible mechanisms suggested are a structural defect in the glomerular basement membrane (Bianchi), a reduction in the number of nephrons and therefore the filtering area (Brenner) or a functional heterogeneity of the nephrons (Sealey and Laragh). Na-K ATPase inhibition, demonstrated in hypertensive patients or those sensitive to hypertension (Garay), could be the common consequence.

32. Eaton S.B., Konner M., Shostak M. Stone-agers in the fast lane: chronic degenerative diseases in evolutionary perspective. *Am J Med* 1988; 84: 739-749.

33. Another cliché is that of the unemployed immigrant whose diet is a little heavier and contains a little more salt than it did in his homeland, victim of urban stress and who could recover "better health" by returning to a simpler and more sober lifestyle.

Studies of migrants have shown that a change of environment is not necessarily without consequence. But the presence of hypertension in non-migrant populations as well as the maintenance of a normal blood pressure in certain migrant populations clearly indicates that genetic constitution can remain the overriding factor despite changes in the environment. Likewise, the inhabitants of large Western cities with their reputedly harmful environments are fortunately not all hypertensive [34]!

If we recognise that hypertension is the end result of the interaction between genetic predisposition to intermediate phenotypes that can promote hypertension on the one hand, and complex interrelated environmental factors on the other, then perhaps it is appropriate to go back and ponder one of the initial questions raised. Why is it, for example, that country people have a low prevalence of hypertension in their native environment and why does it increase when the environment changes ? The role of changes in dietary habits has been discussed at length. Could this mean that one of the ultimate purposes of tradition and culture is to protect the members of a community, with their original genetic make-up, against the devastating influences of outside intervention ? Viewed in this light, each community can be considered to have acquired its own specific "adaptive wisdom". If this is true, the millenia that have elapsed since the days of our hunter-gatherer ancestors would be of scant importance. The important factors would be the large scale migrations of recent history which upset the delicate equilibria built up and painstakingly maintained until that time.

34. The widespread myth of an unhealthy industrial society and the healthy country air has no scientific basis. The fact is that never in the history of humanity has life expectancy been so long and the record holders are the inhabitants of the Western nations.

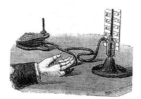

Society under pressure: stress, inequalities and economic pressures

"And so together they went to consult their doctor. "It's your blood pressure" he told them. The word made an impression on him, but all things considered this new obsession was quite a timely occurrence. He had been worrying himself sick for so many years about not being able to meet the payments on his mortgage that all of a sudden there was a sort of free place in the maze of anxieties which had held him captive in fervent apprehension for forty years. Now that his doctor had drawn attention to his blood pressure, he could lie awake at night listening to his blood pressure beating against the pillow. He could even get up to feel his pulse, standing there motionless next to the bed for hours feeling his entire body gently quiver with each heart beat. "This is surely death", he told himself. He had always been afraid of life, but at least now he had something on which to crystallise his fear — his blood pressure — as he had done for the past forty years worrying about not being able to pay off the mortgage on his house".

Louis Ferdinand Celine, 1952
Voyage au bout de la nuit
(A voyage to the end of the night)

Like most diseases, hypertension manifests itself differently according to the influence of sociological parameters such as level of education, status of employment, income or what is generally called "stress" [1]. The multifactorial nature of elevated blood pressure makes an aetiological approach extremely difficult so that we will limit this discussion to epidemiological observation.

1. These factors have also been implicated in the prevalence of such diseases as tuberculosis and cancer.

MODERN CIVILISATION UNDER PRESSURE

The interrelationships between emotivity and blood pressure did not escape the early investigators such as Potain or Riva-Rocci [2]. Having made this observation, physicians conceived the existence of blood pressure variations related to the psyche and many examples could be cited of articles which, as far back as 1910, alluded to the *"oscillations of the systolic blood pressure under the influence of psychic factors"* [3].

2. See chapter 1 — Measuring blood pressure.

3. Zabel. *Münch Med Wochenscher*, n° 44, 1910.

But beyond simple measurement lies the temptation to interpret. Here again, the literature is full of conflicting opinions. Some believed that *"hypotension is an objective sign of psychasthenia"* and a drop in blood pressure *"can be considered as a sure sign of the organic nature of psychasthenia"* [4]. Others maintained that a rise of blood pressure is secondary to "nervousness". There is an evident closeness of meaning between the words "stress" and "pressure" (both words are taken from the language of the physicists) which has fostered both individual and collective interpretations (hypertension is a disease of "nerves", but also a disease of "civilisation"). In 1957, a certain Doctor René Lacroix, in a popular medical book superbly entitled *Protect your blood pressure. Arterial hypertension - a disease of civilisation*, leaves no room for doubt: *"Modern life is essentially vasoconstrictive. It induces a narrowing of the blood vessels with spasms which is the very mechanism of arterial hypertension. Modern life is essentially hypertensive"*. There have been any number of such scientific or pseudo-scientific statements, depending on where they are published, made over the past 100 years and many other examples can be found in areas other than hypertension. According to this concept, the real culprits responsible for hypertension are sociological conditions such as noise, violence, poverty, unemployment or alcoholism, and there have been attempts to equate the level of tension in society with the readings shown by the sphygmomanometer. This is a very old phenomenon which will no doubt be analysed by historians and sociologists who have not yet devoted sufficient attention to cardiovascular diseases [5].

STRESS AND HYPERTENSION: AN EPIDEMIOLOGICAL APPROACH TO A POORLY DEFINED ENTITY

The stress response is largely mediated through the sympathetic nervous system and it is not surprising, therefore, that cardiovascular physiology and stress are intimately linked. The idea that an elevation of blood pressure can simply be caused by the constraints of daily life, an emotional situation or simply by a task perceived as being aggressive is extremely widespread. According to this view, hypertension is simply the consequence of the aggression of a vulnerable subject by society.

This concept would be damaging if it led to the denial of a physiopathological disease process and claimed that hypertension resulted exclusively from the effect of external factors. In the past, tranquillisers were too often used as anti-hypertensive agents (with little effect). Today it is well established that stress (with all the vagueness that the word conveys) alone cannot cause chronic hypertension. It is simply one of the risk factors involved in a multifactorial disease. In contrast, it is true that hypertension is very often accompanied by an abnormal reaction to stress [6].

4. Crouzon O. De la valeur de l'hypotension artérielle comme signe objectif de la psychasthénie (On the value of arterial hypotension as an objective sign of psychasthenia). *Soc Méd Hôpit*, March 26 1915.

5. Postel-Vinay N. L'hypertension artérielle: un chantier de travail pour l'historien ? (Arterial hypertension: a testing ground for historians ?). *Cahiers d'histoire*. Lyon CNRS. 1992. Tome XXXVIII, n°3-4, pp. 230-245.

6. An increased pressor response to various laboratory stimuli such as resolving simple arithmetic problems, video games or psychological tests is well known in hypertensive subjects and in normotensive high-risk subjects (family history).

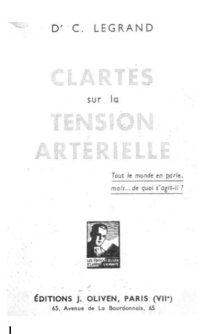

1

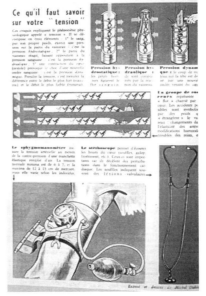

2

Informing the public about the dangers of hypertension

Information campaigns about the dangers of hypertension really took off in the 1960s. But already in 1939, the French public was discovering a book entitled "Clarifying blood pressure" (*figure 1*). Its preface stated: "*The popularisation of a medical instrument or method almost always leads to excess and these excesses need to be corrected. Blood pressure has now acquired superstar status. Everyone is talking about it, in the towns, the countryside, in cafés and factories, without really knowing what they are talking about. Even worse, in the past few months, empirics have sprung up in shops, exhibitions and even on street corners, offering to measure the blood pressure of passers-by. I will show that this innovation is not only imprudent but often fraudulent*".

In 1944 the Saturday Evening Post published an article entitled: "*Killer number one*". In 1952, the New York Daily Mirror referred to hypertension as "*public enemy n°1*" and devoted its front page to the discovery of hexamethonium under the title "Drug aids high blood pressure". In France, the popular scientific press did not remain indifferent. The magazine "*Science et Vie*" (Science and Life) published an article in 1956 explaining "*What you need to know about your blood pressure*" (*figure 2*). In another popular book published in 1957 and entitled "*Protect your blood pressure*" (*figure 3*) we learn that "*hypertension is a disease of civilisation*", a claim that originated in the 1930s. For over half a century now, the general public has been alerted to the problems of hypertension through government agencies, committees or societies, private companies or the media. Many recent surveys have attempted to evaluate the impact of these campaigns but without much success. It would be interesting to complement these surveys with a sociological and historical enquiry like the one recently undertaken for anticancer campaigns. Beyond the strictly medical aspects, it would be of interest to have more information on how the campaigns were organised, how they were financed and the extent of their impact on society.

3

One approach to this question has been to define the so-called "hypertensive personality". The "borderline" hypertensive patient is often young, very emotional and anxious [7]. This emotional instability is associated with an increased sympathetic response (tachycardia, sweating, tremor, blushing) and an increase in plasma catecholamine levels.

Apart from this characteristic full-blown profile, well known to clinicians, it is difficult to define a personality on the basis of classification criteria that are reliable enough to correlate with objective measurable parameters [8]. This difficulty is reflected in the multitude of methods, scales and classification systems that have been used. The hypertensive personality traits most often quoted are anxiety and suppressed aggression. These traits correlate closely with the response to stress in statistical series [9]. These legendary and somewhat fragile data have nevertheless been substantiated by less biased longitudinal studies [10].

While the majority of studies have not shown a relationship between hypertension and what might be termed a "vital events" score, several studies have shown an increased incidence of hypertension in the unemployed. The loss of employment is indisputably associated with increased morbidity and mortality, largely due to cardiovascular causes [11].

The social environment also plays a role. In Detroit for example, the prevalence of hypertension has been reported to be 2.5 times higher amongst the inhabitants of "rough" neighbourhoods than in the "calmer" middle to upper class suburbs. It must be remembered of course that stress is by no means the only factor differentiating these two types of populations. Amongst airport employees, hypertension has been reported to affect air traffic controllers to a greater degree than people employed in less "risky" positions whose stress levels are assumed to be lower. Noise levels in the work environment have also been accused of promoting hypertension [12].

In the face of this evidence, there is a tendency to incriminate stress in many situations where an unusually high incidence of hypertension is observed. The interpretations are sometimes a bit far-fetched. For example, to explain the atypical distribution of hypertension on an island claimed by both Taiwan and mainland China, a recent study incriminated war-related stress and a "hard-line" political regime. Since measurement became possible, preoccupation with blood pressure has accompanied the events of the moment. During World War I, physicians even took their sphygmomanometers with them into the trenches. *"Front-line soldiers, 100 to 150 metres from the enemy, tended to have lower systolic and diastolic pressures than soldiers in*

7. The profile is less clear-cut in overt hypertension, where the patient is usually older and with lower catecholamine levels than the younger subject.

8. It has been suggested that hypertensive patients with personality traits such as suppressed aggression and idealisation of social behaviour have an increased coronary risk.

9. Consoli S.M. Approche psychosomatique de l'hypertension artérielle (Psychosomatic approach to hypertension). *Encyclopédie médico-chirurgicale.* 11302 C10, 3-1990.

10. Perini C., Müller F.B., Bühler F.R. Suppressed aggression accelerates early development of essential hypertension. *J Hyperten* 1991; 9: 499-503.

11. Brackbill et al. recently reported a study on 100,000 subjects questioned by telephone (random numbers) throughout the United States. Overall, the relative risk of hypertension was 1.7 (1.4 - 2.1) for people who had been unemployed for a year or more. The risk was highest for men with a low level of education (3.3 with a range of 2.1 to 5.2). Brackbill R.M., Siegel P.Z., Ackerman S.P. Self-reported hypertension among unemployed people in the United States. *Brit Med J* 1995; 310: 568.

12. Lang et al. studied 7, 900 subjects living in the Paris area. Systolic blood pressure was higher in subjects exposed to noise levels above 85 dB but this difference was no longer statistically significant after adjusting for confounding variables such as age and alcohol consumption. In contrast, the prevalence of hypertension increased with the duration of exposure from 8.2% for exposure lasting less than 20 years to 19% between 20 and 24 years and 37.8% beyond 24 years. After adjusting for other factors, the

the second or third lines [...]. It would appear that regular measurement of blood pressure reflects objectively the state of fatigue and resistance of a battalion" [13]. The measurement of biological parameters and the significance attached to them were sometimes taken to ideological excess — but that is another story. Not all the early observers were quite so rash. Laubry, for example, in 1917, denounced the "*imperturbable dogmatism of the German authors who supported functional tests based on blood pressure measurement*". Laubry denied accusations of "*systematic criticism of sphygmomanometry*". He argued for a more cautious approach in interpreting certain results: "*We have not observed in the soldiers under our command any characteristic response or special features not found in other healthy individuals.*

relative risk associated with noise exposure lasting 25 years or more was 2.59 (0.96 - 6.99). Other studies in other countries have shown similar results. Lang T. Fouriaud C., Jacquinet-Salord M.C. Length of occupational noise exposure and blood pressure. *Int Arch Occup Environ Health* 1992; 63: 369-72.

13. Ménard P. Sur la pression artérielle et le pouls chez le soldat dans les tranchées (Blood pressure and pulse rates of soldiers in the trenches). *Acad méd*, October 17th, 1916.

Table 1

Sociocultural and economic factors promoting hypertension (according to S.G. Rostand)

Changes in social structure

Unrestrained urbanisation and westernisation

Geographical changes
    Migration to urban areas
    Migration to another continent

Environmental changes

Increase in stress
    Changes in family structure
    Interethnic conflict, changes in values

Socio-economic disturbances
    Change in occupational status
    Unemployment
    Loss of income
    Insufficient or poorly adapted level of education
    Difficult access to health services

Biological changes
    Changes in the level of activity
    Changes in exposure to ultraviolet rays, vitamin D deficiency
    Changes in diet (sodium, potassium, fatty acids)
    Weight gain (diabetes, insulin resistance, atheroma)

This negative conclusion is not surprising when one considers that blood pressure regulation is dependent on multiple factors of mechanical, nervous, cardiac, vasomotor, central or peripheral origin which complement each other and can easily conceal any given deficiency. This very complexity should deter us from hasty conclusions and make us wary of creating categories in which different types of patients, for example those with normal and abnormal vasomotor function, would be artificially grouped" [14].

STANDARD OF LIVING: DOES BLOOD PRESSURE RISE WHEN INCOME DROPS?

Epidemiological studies have demonstrated an inverse correlation between level of education, income and blood pressure. There is widespread belief, already mentioned in the literature of the 1920s, that people at the managerial level pay a heavy tribute to hypertension. In fact, there are numerous studies showing that the prevalence of hypertension is inversely related with socio-professional status. In the Hypertension Detection and Follow-up Program, the prevalence of hypertension in Whites was 13.5% for individuals who had been to university versus 23% for those who had remained in school for less than 10 years [15].

In France, death from coronary artery disease over the past 20 years has evolved very differently in different socio-professional groups. There has been a 5-fold decrease in managerial staff (121/million in 1990), whereas the decrease has been less striking in employees (535/million) and in farmers (250/million). A similar pattern has been observed for death resulting from cerebral vascular accidents and for general mortality. Compared to senior managers, the relative risk of death from coronary artery disease or cerebral vascular accidents is 3.50 and 2.93 respectively for employees. The corresponding figures for labourers are 1.78 and 1.70 respectively [16].

Hypertension is less often detected in the lower socio-economic groups [17]. The common feature of these poorly detected groups is the absence of regular health care and the almost exclusive reliance on emergency services. This inequality is not dependent only on income but also on the general ability to "cope with the system".

The difficulties encountered by certain social categories in obtaining information and adequate health care prompted the creation of societies whose aim was to inform the general public about the problems of hypertension. Sporadic programs sprung up, for example to measure people's blood pressure in public places and even in supermarkets. Television and press campaigns were initiated in an attempt to inform the public about the problems of hypertension and its relationship with lifestyle factors. The impact of these campaigns is difficult to evaluate.

14. Laubry C. Variations du rythme cardiaque et la tension artérielle dans l'orthostatisme, l'effort et la fatigue. Leur valeur au point de vue de l'aptitude militaire (variations in cardiac rhythm and blood pressure with orthostatism, exertion and fatigue. Their value from the point of view of aptness for service). *Arch mal coeur et vaisseaux* 1917; 1: 49-65.

15. Hypertension detection and follow-up cooperative group: race, education, and prevalence of hypertension. *Amer J Epidem* 1977; 106: 351-356.

16. Lang T., Ducimetière P. Premature cardio-vascular mortality in France: divergent evolution between social categories from 1970 to 1990. *Int J Epidemiol* 1995; 24: 331-339.

17. The level of detection is lower for example in immigrants than in the indigenous population. In France, 35% of the indigenous population are not aware of their hypertension compared to 63% of immigrants. The unemployed also tend to have lower levels of detection. Lang T. Degoulet P., Ménard J. Socio-economic influences on treatment. In Handbook of hypertension, vol 13: *The management of hypertension.* 1990. F.R. Bühler and J.H. Laragh. Elsevier.

We know that the general level of awareness has increased over time and that a higher proportion of hypertensive patients are now being treated. But there are no doubt negative aspects to these campaigns which have probably increased the number of unwarranted treatments. It would be interesting to undertake a retrospective analysis to elucidate how these campaigns were organised and financed (public or private funds) and what relationship they had with the media and the pharmaceutical industry [18].

Disparities are also observed in regard to compliance with treatment. Statistics from a Paris hospital reveal that the percentage of hypertensive patients lost to follow-up was 22% for underprivileged categories, compared to 16% for senior management level patients. Compliance with medical treatment was estimated to be 57% for labourers and employees versus 73% for managerial level individuals. The importance of these factors is aptly illustrated in the HDFP study [19]. In the "stepped care" group, subjected to routine control of blood pressure, there was no difference in mortality according to social category. This was not the case in the "referred care" group, treated on a "by request" basis.

MANAGED CARE OF HYPERTENSION: FROM MEDICINE TO ECONOMICS

Environmental and socio-cultural factors can influence the prevalence of hypertension as we have seen. Society attempts to counter these effects through public programs of information, screening and treatment. This undertaking goes far beyond the purely medical and scientific aspects of the past hundred years to raise a totally new issue: that of cost. Medicine today is increasingly concerned with economic issues which have important sociological and political repercussions. The intrusion of socio-economic factors into medical practice affects all areas of medicine and is by no means confined to hypertension. But if one takes into account the fact that over half the elderly population has a blood pressure above the accepted norm [20], that cardiovascular disease remains a major cause of morbidity and mortality in the Western world and that cardiovascular medicine ranks high amongst the priorities of the pharmaceutical industry, it is clear that the impact of socio-economic factors on hypertension is considerable.

The management of hypertension includes recommendations concerning lifestyle and diet, visits to the doctor, sometimes hospitalisation, laboratory tests and radiological and other imaging techniques, all of which often culminate in a drug prescription. In the early 20th century, when drug manufacturing was becoming an industrial process, the pharmaceutical industry soon realised that vascular diseases represented a substantial market [21].

18. A socio-historical study on anti-cancer campaigns has recently been completed by Patrice Pinell in France. This work could serve as a model for campaigns on hypertension.

19. Hypertension detection and follow-up program cooperative group: educational level and 5-year all-cause mortality in the hypertension detection and follow-up program. *Hypertension* 1987; 9: 641-646

20. See chapter 5 — The question of norms.

21. It is of interest to note that in its very first year (1908), the French medical journal *"Archives des maladies du coeur, des vaisseaux et du sang"* (Archives of diseases of the heart, vessels and blood) devoted one third of its pages to drug advertising. Drugs against arteriosclerosis and "hypotensive" agents (including mistletoe-based preparations and iodinated products) were well represented.

In 1990, health care expediture accounted for 12% of the GNP in the United States (compared to around 8% in European countries). In a country like France, the pharmaceutical sector represents 17% of the total health care budget, i.e. 1.4% of GNP [22]. These percentages are continually on the rise and sooner or later, a limit will have to be imposed. C. Le Pen, a health economist, estimates the annual cost of cardiovascular diseases in France to be around $7 billion, of which $3.4 to 5.4 billion is directly attributable to hypertension-related disorders.

Immediately after the Second World War, considerable sums were invested to develop new antihypertensive agents. The energy which was — and still is — expended to promote these drugs is commensurate with the expected financial rewards. Since the 1970s, the pharmaceutical industry has been successful in developing valuable drugs for hypertensive patients which have transformed medical practice and radically modified prescribing habits [23]. Even medical publishing and scientific meetings have been influenced to an extent that has had an impact on fundamental scientific questions [24]. The difficulties encountered today by most countries in balancing their health budgets means that medical practice is being urged to save money. The purely scientific aspects of medicine will probably not emerge unscathed from this new orientation which, of course, does not apply only to hypertension.

In a recent edition of a book on hypertension [25], Kaplan notes that unrestrained enthusiasm for early and aggressive drug therapy began in the 1970s. Today in the United States the treatment of hypertension is the number one motive for medical consultation and drug prescription. As a consequence, 30% of Americans aged 55 to 64 are on antihypertensive medications. The proportion rises to 40% between the ages of 65 and 74 and it is likely that these figures are still increasing.

The need for an ever-increasing number of patients to be taking antihypertensive drugs can be seriously questioned and there is every reason to believe that a large number of patients is being treated irrationally without a proper diagnosis of permanent hypertension. This situation raises two important issues. The first is strictly medical and has to do with good clinical practice. Which measurement methods should be used to avoid overdiagnosing hypertension ? What is the true efficacy of mass treatment of hypertension ? The second issue is an economic one. In this context, "too much drug" no longer signifies toxicity, but economic wastage. The two issues are often confused in the literature [26] because financial considerations often encroach on the scientific aspects and vice-versa.

The problem of the choice of a first-line drug is illustrative in this regard. In the evolving history of drug development, as new drugs became available, doctors' prescriptions understandably changed. With each change two distinct aspects had to be considered. The first was the new

22. Tessier P. *Les médicaments: l'avenir pour l'homme?* (Pharmaceuticals: man's future?) 1991; Editions du Rocher, Paris.

23. See chapter 4 — Treating hypertension.

24. Promotional spending by the pharmaceutical industry rose from $6 million in 1975 to $86 million in 1988. Out of 283 sponsored symposia published in the international medical press, 45% were published by only 3 journals, two of which dealt with cardiovascular medicine (*American Heart Journal* and the *American Journal of Cardiology*). Out of 625 sponsored symposia analysed by Bero et al., 42% had a single sponsor. Out of 161 symposia dealing with a single compound, in 86 cases the compound was a cardiovascular one (compared to 18 antibotics and 12 anti-inflammatory compounds). Bero et al. pointed out that for special supplements to journals sponsored by the pharmaceutical industry, the usual peer-review system was not often applied. Bero L.A., Galbraith P.A., Drumond Rennie B.A. The publication of sponsored symposiums in medical journals. *N Engl J Med* 1992; 327: 1135-1140.

25. Kaplan N.M. *Clinical hypertension.* Sixth ed. 1994. Williams & Wilkins, Baltimore.

26. For more on the debate surrounding the management of hypertension, see chapter 7 — Yesterday's sufferers, today's patients.

drug's efficacy and the advantages it provided for patients. The second aspect was its cost for society. A gradual transition is occurring in the use of antihypertensive drugs. The older, cheaper drugs (diuretics and beta-blockers) are being replaced by the newer, more expensive drugs (ACE inhibitors and calcium channel blockers).

In the United States for example, where diuretics were well established as first-line drugs, this class has recently been supplanted in a number of prescriptions by the calcium channel blockers. The cost of one month of treatment with a generic preparation of hydrochlorothiazide is $0.27 compared to $39 for a calcium channel blocker [27].

27. Strasser T. Relative costs of anti-hypertensive drug treatment. *J Hum Hypertens* 1992; 6: 489-94.

Like drugs, investigational techniques also face a financial-scientific dilemma as costs escalate. Depending on the physician's choice and the clinical situation, the work-up of a hypertensive patient can vary considerably in cost. Twenty-four-hour blood pressure recordings, cardiac ultrasound and other technological innovations are causing costs to escalate, thereby creating new potential sources of conflict between clinical and economic requisites.

In an attempt to resolve these issues, studies on "cost-effectiveness" were undertaken. The cost, for example, of a "quality-adjusted life year" saved by antihypertensive treatment is estimated to be $1,748 and the gain in life-expectancy from such treatment is anywhere from 1 to 5 years depending on the baseline blood pressure [28]. This type of estimation bears little resemblance to clinical reality and the variations from one study to another are quite substantial. A number of mathematical models, which appear somewhat surrealistic to clinicians, have been proposed to quantify this non-measurable parameter.

28. Maynard A. The economics of hypertension control: some basic issues. *J Hum Hypertens* 1992; 6: 417-420.

29. Kawachi I., Malcolm L.A. Cost-effectiveness of treating mild to moderate hypertension: a reappraisal. *J Hypertens* 1991; 9: 199-208.

Calculating the cost/benefit ratio of treatment
(from Kawachi et al [29])

$$\frac{C}{B} = \frac{(\Delta C_{RX} + \Delta C_{SE} - \Delta C_{morb})}{(\Delta Y_{LE} - \Delta Y_{SE} + \Delta Y_{morb})}$$

C = net cost of treatment
B = net benefit of treatment
ΔC_{RX} = direct cost of treatment
ΔC_{SE} = cost of treating side-effects
ΔC_{morb} = saving achieved by preventing complications
ΔY_{LE} = increase in life-expectancy resulting from treatment
ΔY_{SE} = decrease in life-expectancy resulting from side-effects
ΔY_{morb} = benefit in terms of quality of life resulting from the prevention of complications

These models tell us that it is more "cost-effective" to treat severe hypertension than to treat mild hypertension and that treating an elderly patient is more cost-effective than treating a young patient. Indeed, it makes sense, without having to resort to mathematics, that treating a patient with a short-term risk will also procure an advantage in the short term, with less years of treatment required. A recent study even considered that it was not cost-effective to use drug treatment in mild to moderate hypertension and suggested that a non-pharmacological strategy needed to be devised in such cases [29].

HYPERTENSION AND POLITICS

In the face of these budgetary considerations how are governments reacting ? Ménard talks metaphorically about "*oil and water*" with regard to the medical and political aspects. Confronted with conflicting interests, health authorities are turning to expert committees in order to formulate pseudo-scientific arguments to justify the obvious observation that the less expensive a drug, the higher the quality/cost ratio of treatment [30]. These committees publish adeptly prepared guidelines based on indisputable clinical and epidemiological data to end up with strategies based essentially on economic considerations. Thus, the recommendations of the WHO - International Society of Hypertension, or the guidelines of the Joint National Committee, have been hotly debated [31]. These recommendations have all rightly emphasised the need for an irrefutable diagnosis of moderate hypertension before initiating treatment. They have also stressed the importance of a non-drug, lifestyle modification approach for several months in order to select those patients who really need drug therapy. This is simply common sense, but it certainly is worthwhile including them in the guidelines to remind doctors of their importance and give them "official" status. More controversial, particularly in the fifth report of the Joint National Committee, is the recommendation for the preferential use of the cheaper diuretics and betablockers as first-line agents, pending adequate evidence (increasingly difficult to obtain) that the more expensive drugs have any advantage in terms of morbidity. These recommendations have been criticised and Ménard comments on the fifth JNC report by saying: "*The recommendation to prescribe the cheapest drug is a denial of both scientific progress and medical art*". Indeed, there is evidence to suggest that angiotensin converting enzyme inhibitors do have advantages, not only in terms of patient acceptability and quality of life, but probably also in terms of cardiac, vascular and renal protection. Will we have to deny patients these benefits for years while we wait for the results of hypothetical mortality studies? Are such recommendations not contrary to the prospects for "personalising treatment"?

In the midst of this debate, how can general practictioners, the main prescribers of antihypertensive drugs, find their way ? They are trapped

30. Ménard J. Oil and Water ? Economic advantage and biomedical progress do not mix well in a government guidelines committee. *Am J Hypertens* 1994; 7: 877-885.

31. Subcommittee of WHO/ISH Mild Hypertension Liaison Committee: Summary of 1993 World Health Organisation-International Society of Hypertension guidelines for the management of mild hypertension. *Brit Med J* 1993; 307: 1541-1546.
Joint National Committee on detection, evaluation and treatment of high blood pressure. Fifth report. *Arch Int Med* 1993; 153: 154-183.

between the pressure of pharmaceutical advertising which constantly reminds them that increasingly effective drugs are available, and official bodies which encourage them to be more economical in their prescribing. Both parties refer to the conclusions of their "experts" which overwhelm the modest practitioners trying to do their best for their patients. The confusion of doctors faced with these recent developments in hypertension is a totally new facet of the impact of contemporary society on hypertension and its treatment. A new page in the history of hypertension is being written.

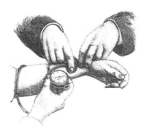

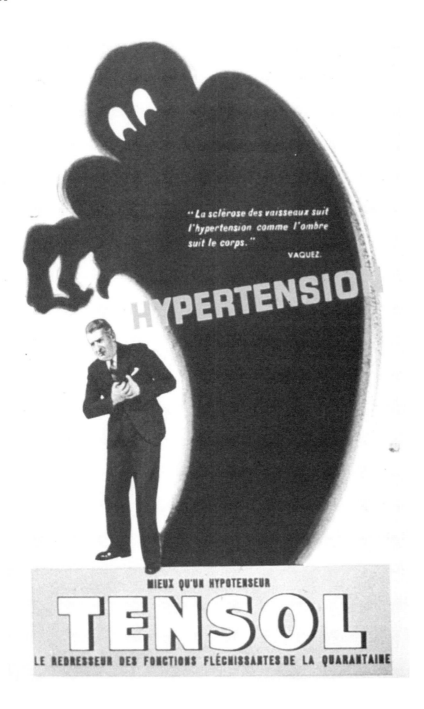

Advertisement in the French medical press (1950s)

The advertisement quotes Vaquez: "Sclerosis of the vessels follows hypertension like a shadow follows the body". It also claims: "TENSOL is more than a hyptensive agent — it restores the declining functions of middle-age".

7

YESTERDAY'S SUFFERERS
AND TODAY'S PATIENTS

Towards the disappearance of symptoms

"It is your art itself that intrigues me. I wonder how you know, and what a mind you must have to be able to speak to me the way you did just a while ago, so truthfully and unpresumptuously, when you said, or rather predicted, that at daybreak tomorrow I would feel better and be cured. I marvel at what you must be, you and your medicine, to obtain from my nature this prophetic spirit capable of sensing the promise of recovery. Why does this body of mine confide in you and not in me? To me it speaks only of hardship, pain and fatigue, as if it were abusing me to express its displeasure. It speaks to my soul as to an animal, led without explanation but only with violence and outrage. But to you it conveys clearly what it wants, what it does not want and the whys and wherefores of its state. How strange it is that you should know infinitely more than I about myself, and that I should be so transparent to the light of your knowledge, whereas unto myself I am but obscurity and impenetrability".

Paul Valéry [1]
Socrate et son médecin (Socrates and his physician)

[1]. Paul Valéry: French novelist 1847-1945.

Vivid historic descriptions of patients suffering from apoplexy, Bright's disease or malignant hypertension testify to the severe nature of the symptoms of hypertensive patients at the turn of the century. In the period 1890-1920, hypertensive patients were often those with renal failure and cardiac failure in whom atherosclerosis had taken a heavy toll for many years. They were breathless, tired and complained of headache and dizziness. Their arteries were rigid (or "senile" as they were described at the time), their heart markedly enlarged, their fundi abnormal and their kidneys secreted albumin. In a word they were severely ill and generally confined to hospital. *"Dyspnoea is the fifth act of hypertension"* wrote Allbutt in 1915 [2], by which he was probably referring to the cardiac failure of hypertensive patients.

As early as 1905-1910, a few perceptive physicians realised that hypertension could also affect less symptomatic patients, but it was not

[2]. Allbutt C. Diseases of the arteries including angina pectoris. London 1915, vol. 1, p. 381; vol. 2, p. 61. Cited by Ayman. Ayman D., Pratt J., Nature of the symptoms associated with essential hypertension. *Arch Int Med* 1931;47: 675-687.

until after 1920 that measurement of blood pressure started to become popular. It was then discovered that there was such a thing as an asymptomatic hypertensive patient. But in fact there were not very many of them for at least three reasons. First, the absence of any effective form of therapy meant that blood pressure was not controlled in the majority of cases. Second, routine measurement of blood pressure remained confined to insurance company physicians and last, since hypertension was not recognised as a risk factor, there was no established epidemiological definition of it. Between the two world wars, the management of hypertension was viewed in the traditional medical setting of a patient coming to see his doctor to seek relief from some symptom. The objective was to relieve the patient of his headaches, dizziness or other "circulatory disturbances". The approach was to diagnose and to relieve — not to prevent.

THE AGE OF SYMPTOMS

Historically, it is difficult to have a clear idea of how important the symptoms of hypertension were considered to be, but no doubt they were the major component of the disease in the first half of this century. This is clearly reflected in a an article by Ayman and Pratt entitled *Nature of the symptoms associated with essential hypertension* published in 1931 [3]. According to many authors cited by Ayman, hypertension was responsible for two types of manifestations — early and late-onset. The early signs were headaches, nervousness, fatigability, irritability and dizziness, sometimes associated with "premonitory signs" such as cyanosis of the extremities. This symptom-based approach was so dominant that some authors thought they could even recognise *"manometrically normal hypertension"* by the presence of *"vasomotor disturbances, flushing, epistaxis, migraine or cold, sweaty and cyanotic hands"*! Ayman opposed this view, but it is very revealing of the imprecise significance of the actual blood pressure readings at the time.

In order to form his own opinion about the symptoms of hypertension, Ayman decided to screen 100 "unselected" hypertensive patients. He defined a hypertensive patient as one whose systolic blood pressure had exceeded 160 mmHg on several occasions but who had no renal lesions (Ayman gives no further information on the method of measurement he used). The patients were screened for 25 distinct symptoms which proved to be very prevalent: 72% of the subjects had headaches, 65% complained of fatigue, 54% exhibited "localised flushes", 30% reported gastric discomfort and 28% complained of a loss of appetite. Ayman hit upon the idea of comparing these symptoms to those of "psychoneuroses" and observed that *"the early symptoms of arterial hypertension cannot be distinguished from those of psychoneurosis"*. He concluded his study in these terms: *"While it seems reasonable to conclude that the early*

3. Ayman D., Pratt J. Nature of the symptoms associated with essential hypertension. *Arch Int Med.* 1931; 47: 675-687.

The symptoms of hypertension viewed by Theodore C. Janeway in 1913

1. The most prominent symptoms associated with high blood pressure are circulatory rather than renal. The disease underlying high arterial pressure is predominantly a disease of the circulatory system, and is best designated hypertensive cardiovascular disease, either primary, or secondary when preceded by an inflammatory nephritis.

2. Death in this type of cardiovascular disease, among patients in private practice, occurs in the following ways, arranged in the order of their frequency: first, by gradual cardiac insufficiency; second, with uremic symptoms; third, by apoplexy; fourth, from some complicating acute infection; fifth, in an attack of angina pectoris; sixth, from purely accidental and unrelated causes; seventh, in a paroxysm of acute edema of the lungs; eight, after the manner of cachexia.

3. The early symptoms associated with hypertensive cardiovascular disease have an important prognostic significance which can be utilized therapeutically, particularly for the institution of safeguarding treatment.

4. The early occurrence of symptoms of myocardial weakness, especially dyspnea, indicates a more than 50 per cent probability of an eventual death by cardiac insufficiency. In these patients, to safeguard the heart is the main therapeutic indication.

5. The early occurrence of anginoid pain on exertion does not indicate a probability of death in an anginal paroxysm for more than one-third of the patients. It does indicate a probable cardiac death of some type. The therapeutic indications here are similar to the foregoing, except as modified by the existence of syphilitic aortitis. Anginal attacks as compared with other cardiac symptoms do not materially affect the expectancy of life.

6. Polyuria, particularly if nocturnal, indicates the probability of a uremic death for more than 50 per cent of the patients. It is not essential to safeguard the heart in these patients, unless associated cardiac symptoms exist.

7. Headache, especially that heretofore described as typical, indicates the probability of a uremic death for more than 50 per cent of the patients, and of the death from apoplexy for a considerable number of the remainder. The therapeutic indications are similar to those of polyuria.

8. Loss of flesh, if marked and progressive, is a symptom of bad prognostic import.

From: A clinical study of hypertensive cardiovascular disease. Theodore C. Janeway. *Archives of Internal Medicine*, 1913; 12: 755-798.

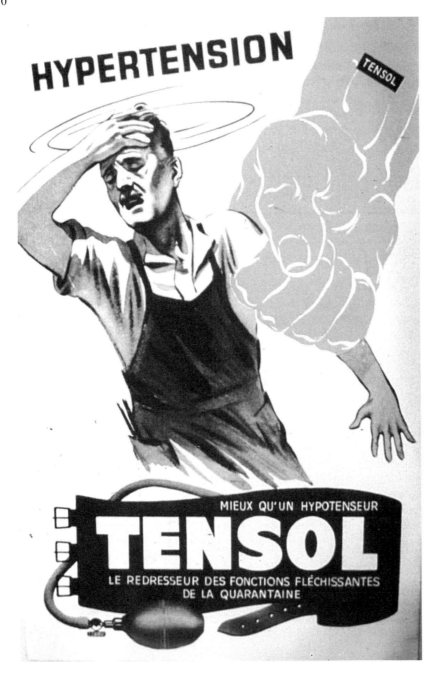

Advertisement in the French medical press (1950s)

While, the advertisement depicts a patient with symptomatic hypertension, the slogan makes false promises: "TENSOL is more than a hypotensive agent — it restores the declining functions of middle-age".

symptoms associated with essential hypertension are probably of psychic origin, the fundamental mechanism is not clear. Constitutional influences, endocrine products and possibly other factors may contribute to lessen the hypertensive patient's psychic capacity for withstanding the stress and strain of life".

THE LOGIC OF PREVENTION:
A STEP TOWARDS "NORMALITY"

In the decade 1950-1960, the lessons from the Framingham study and the progress made in pharmacology began to stir up the debate on mass screening. The logic of prevention, which had appeared timidly ten or twenty years earlier, began to gain momentum and doctors started taking a newly found interest in the asymptomatic hypertensive patient. Patients with mild hypertension who now needed prevention of the development of complications, suddenly found themselves to be in the majority, while severely hypertensive patients (who needed to be treated) quickly became a minority. This new distribution of the patient population brought with it changes in the way patients were diagnosed, followed-up and treated. Measuring blood pressure, taking x-rays and prescribing drugs remained important, but other investigations were added to the list and became more refined since what was now being sought was not quite so overt. Tests were being done earlier in the natural history of hypertension, so it was no surprise to find that they were increasingly close to "normal".

In this regard, a detailed history of the study of the heart in hypertension is an excellent illustration of the changes that have occurred in the management of patients. As we will see, in a century of hypertension the heart gradually diminished in size as doctors increasingly turned their attention to the beginnings of the cardiovascular disease process. These transformations, which are by no means particular to hypertension, reflect the evolution of the modern doctor-patient relationship in which the symptom loses some of its importance and the statistical analysis of laboratory tests becomes dominant.

THE EXAMPLE OF LEFT VENTRICULAR HYPERTROPHY:
FROM THE SCALPEL TO ULTRASOUND

The example of ideas surrounding left ventricular hypertrophy in hypertension aptly illustrates the gradual changes that occurred in the management of patients with hypertension.

Left ventricular hypertrophy was not invented by the specialists of hypertension — far from it. It was recognised for the first time in the 17th century when scientists adopted a quantitative and dynamic view of the human body after William Harvey described the heart as a pump and showed how the circulatory system worked [4].

4. *Exercitatio anatomica de motu cordis et sanguinis in animalibus* (Anatomical exercises on the movement of the heart and blood of animals). William Harvey, Frankfurt, 1628.

From then on, physiologists wondered about the laws that regulated blood flow, while the anatomists studied organ alterations in an attempt to determine the causes of death. In 1761, Morgagni published his innovative work which attempted to correlate symptoms observed during life, with anatomical lesions found in the cadaver [5]. He noted that the heart was "dilated" (aneurysms) or "ossified" (atheroma). Attempts were made to explain these abnormalities, and a century later Sénac remarked that "*the cavities of the heart are often distended when blood has been driven there by violent exertion*" and he observed that "*the volume of the heart may increase or decrease*" [6]. By doing autopsies, he was able to study aneurysms, polyps and pericardial effusions. Amongst the causes of cardiac "*dilatation*" he recognised the contribution of the "*mass and the force of the blood*". He distinguished between the dilatation of the atria and that of the left ventricle and his perspicacity led him to ponder on "*the force of the dilated heart*". He suspected that the fibres of the heart could become stronger by "*growing like the muscles of a child*" [7]. In the 18th century, anatomical lesions of the heart responsible for disease began to be suspected well before the concept of hypertension or Starling's laws and even before, doctors were performing more than a semblance of clinical examination.

In the 19th century, the new anatomico-clinical method, correlating autopsy findings with clinical symptoms, provided doctors with a means of recognising heart disease in patients, not simply in cadavers. Corvisart rediscovered percussion and Laënnec invented auscultation, and so it became possible to feel and to listen to the heart, which began to disclose its secrets. Its murmurs revealed valvular alterations de vivo, and its dullness on percussion betrayed an aneurysm or an effusion. At the turn of the 19th century, Corvisart knew how to distinguish "*simple, eccentric or concentric hypertrophy*". Cardiac enlargement was now recognisable by specific clinical signs and could be diagnosed at the bedside [8]. Different types of hypertrophy were described: those resulting from valve disease, but also the essential hypertrophies of heavy manual labourers and pregnant women, and the enlarged hearts of "fatty degeneration" [9]. On the other side of the English channel, Richard Bright remarked that out of 100 deaths in patients with albuminuria, "*the variable state of the heart is most noteworthy*" and he stressed the frequency of cardiac enlargement in patients with renal failure.

In 1806, Corvisart published his *Essay on diseases and organic lesions of the heart and great vessels* in which he classified cardiac enlargement into two categories which he called "*active and passive aneurysms*". Two years later he translated and analysed at length Auenbrugger's book *A new method for recognising chest diseases by percussion*. This publication popularised percussion in Europe.

On page 651 of the second edition of his book *Diseases of the heart* (1826) Corvisart stated: "*The heart, as well as the other muscles of the human body, may increase in size and strength due to the continuity and above all the energy of its action*".

5. Morgagni G.B. *De sedibus et causis morborum per anatomen indagatis* (The location and causes of disease studied by anatomy). Venice, 1761.

6. Sénac J.-B. *Traité de la structure du coeur, de son action et de ses maladies* (Treatise on the heart, its action and diseases). 1749, book IV, chap. VIII, p. 408.

7. "*Let us examine whether this organ is more active when its size increases. At first glance this should not be the case. Muscle fibres do not increase in number when they are distended. However, it is certain that the heart can work with greater violence. I can conceive of only two causes to account for this increased activity. The walls of the heart are thicker and the mass of blood in the ventricles is much greater. Just as children's muscles become stronger as they grow, so the fibres of the heart increase in strength when the heart enlarges*". Jean-Baptiste Sénac. ibid.

8. In the early 19th century, Corvisart, Laënnec and Bouillaud were familiar with the signs and symptoms of left ventricular hypertrophy.

9. Cited by Michel Peter. *Traité clinique et pratique des maladies du coeur et de la crosse de l'aorte* (Clinical and practical treatise on diseases of the heart and the aortic arch). Paris, 1883.

In his famous *Treatise on mediate auscultation in diseases of the lungs and heart* (Paris 1819), Laënnec reported a case in which the application of his "cylinder" (stethoscope) to a patient's chest, allowed him to make the diagnosis of "*ossification of the mitral valve, mild hypertrophy of the left ventricle, possibly mild ossification of the aortic valve and marked hypertrophy of the right ventricle*". Further on in the book, Laënnec disagreed with Corvisart (who claimed he could diagnose ventricular hypertrophy by feeling the pulse [10]): "*The only sure sign of ventricular dilatation is provided by the stethoscope revealing the loud and clear sound of the heart which can be heard between the fifth and seventh sternal ribs*".

Confronted with the limitations of clinical medicine, doctors in the second half of the 19th century increasingly felt the need for what they called a "diagnostic arsenal". After the stethoscope, a number of new instruments were introduced, such as the pleximeter [11], the speculum or the endoscope. Shortly thereafter, the first laboratory tests made their appearance.

But the investigation of left ventricular hypertrophy by precordial palpation and percussion, as was still practised by Janeway in 1913, remained fairly crude [12]. Of course, no mention was made of electrocardiography which was not performed at the time. In Janeway's series of 437 hypertensive patients, 193 died and the 244 surviving patients had a left ventricular hypertrophy diagnosed clinically by the area of dullness on percussion and the displacement of the apex [13].

The introduction of radiology was a major conceptual leap forward. It enabled anatomical abnormalities to be detected before they gave rise to clinical symptoms. After the discovery of x-rays by Röntgen a century ago (1895), radiography very quickly proved to be of value for the study of the cardiovascular system. Vaquez and Bordet in France were amongst the first to turn their attention to radiology in cardiovascular medicine [14]. Having been a student of Potain, Vaquez had been interested in hypertension and he commented on the presence of left ventricular hypertrophy with remarkable foresight. He understood that the radiological study of the heart revealed the sequence of events in the pathological process. "*We thus see the importance of detecting ventricular hypertrophy in its early stages since its presence alone may reflect hypertension which would not otherwise have been suspected and which, it may be feared, will ultimately cause renal sclerosis. While percussion is ordinarily sufficient to recognise the considerable cardiac enlargement of advanced Bright's disease, it is incapable of detecting the more subtle changes of the early phase. This is precisely the moment when the diagnosis needs to be made. Fortunately, radiology is now available to make up for the deficiencies of clinical investigation in this situation*" [14].

10. Corvisart. ibid. Page 510 of the 2nd edition (1826).

11. The pleximeter, conceived by Piorry (a student of Trousseau) was composed of an ivory plate and a small hammer and was meant to make percussion more sensitive. This technical mediation, not really of much use, was nonetheless valued by certain physicians, and occupied a respectful place amongst the medical instruments of the latter past of the 19th century. Cardiac hypertrophy was thus manifested by an increased area of dullness of the percussed chest.

12. In a series reported in 1913, Theodore C. Janeway (one of the first to describe and quantify the incidence of ventricular hypertrophy in hypertension) mentioned that no radiological investigations had been performed. Evidently he was aware of the importance of radiology in the study of left ventricular hypertrophy, but no doubt because of the recent advent of the technique he did not have access to it.

13. Janeway T.C. A clinical study of hypertensive cardiovascular disease. *Arch Int Med* 1913; 2, 755-798.

14. Vaquez and Bordet. *Le coeur et l'aorte. Etude de radiologie clinique* (The heart and the aorta. Radiological studies in clinical medicine) 1913. Baillière , Paris.

In 1921, in an article entitled *The past, the present and the future of hypertensive patients*, Leconte confirmed the prognostic value of radiological examination of hypertensive patients: "*To assess the alterations of the heart and the aorta before any clinical signs are apparent, radioscopy is the most valuable accessory, one could even say the indispensable complement for the examination of the hypertensive patient*" [15].

ANATOMY BECOMES A PROGNOSTIC TOOL

The myocardium of the hypertensive patient is initially "*camouflaged*" stated Donzelot in the title of his article published in 1922 [16]. He went on to explain that it takes several years for myocardial strain to be expressed clinically: "*As long as the myocardium is capable of compensating for the increase in peripheral resistance through enlargement and a more forceful systole, the two signs that we have studied (left ventricular hypertrophy and a louder second aortic sound) are the only clinical signs of the hypertensive heart. But no matter how long the heart holds up, usually for several years, sooner or later signs of weakness become apparent as the heart, invaded by sclerosis, succumbs to the overload*" [16].

Now aware of this sequence of events, doctors began examining their patients radioscopically at regular intervals to assess the severity of hypertension. By measuring the size of the heart, they attempted to deduce the prognosis. Heitz, in 1927, believed that an accentuation in the curvature of the left border of the heart and the apex was predictive of a serious accident. This new way of looking at the myocardial changes in hypertension, no longer simply to collect anatomical information but to make predictions about the future, was quite a revolution. But was it justified ? The answer to this question was to come from the insurance companies and from the Framingham study.

Between the two world wars, there was growing interest for the epidemiology of non-infectious diseases in Great Britain and in the United Sates, fostered by the development of new statistical and epidemiological methods.

Just after the Second World War, the validity of a quantitative approach to the prognosis in hypertension was established. This was achieved in two fundamentally different, but not contradictory ways. In Europe, doctors recorded the blood pressure of their hypertensive patients which they subsequently correlated with outcome. In the anglo-saxon world more emphasis was put on measuring the blood pressure of healthy individuals who wanted to take out a life insurance policy (or who happened to live in Framingham, Massachusetts). Both approaches quickly led to the firm conclusion that cardiac enlargement was a poor prognostic sign for the hypertensive patient.

15. Leconte. *Le passé, le présent et l'avenir des hypertendus* (The past, the present and the future of hypertensive patients). *Paris médical*, July 2nd, 1921. 11-18.

16. Donzelot. Le coeur camouflé des hypertendus (The camouflaged heart of hypertensive patients). *La Presse médicale* 1922, n° 508.

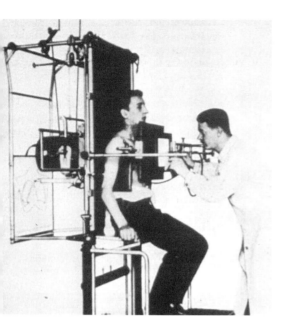

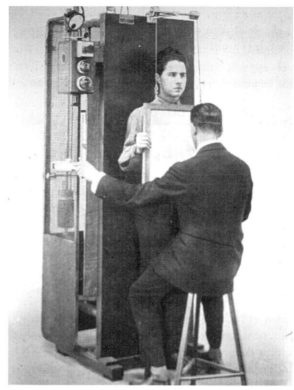

2

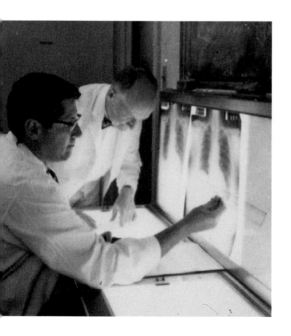

Measuring left ventricular hypertrophy: anatomy as a prognostic tool

Identified in the 18th century, left ventricular hypertrophy is a typical example of how the study of a parameter patterned itself upon the evolution of medical thinking. Initially viewed as an anatomical abnormality, left ventricular hypertrophy gradually became to be considered as a prognostic variable.

In the 19th century, physicians knew how to recognise severe cardiac enlargement by percussing the chest. In the early 20th century, doctors realised the value of following the evolution of left ventricular hypertrophy in hypertensive patients by means of radiological examinations (*figures 1* and *2*). In 1969, the results from the Framingham study confirmed the validity of this approach when they demonstrated that cardiac status was an important prognostic factor (*figure 3*: Dr William Kannel measuring the size of the heart in the Framingham study). Today, echocardiography has supplanted radiology for the follow-up of ventricular hypertrophy in hypertension.

Post-war studies thus confirmed what doctors had suspected for many years. As early as 1913, Vaquez wrote that "*[in certain cases] ventricular hypertrophy is the only pathological phenomenon accompanying hypertension [...]. In fact this sign alone may reveal unsuspected hypertension*" [14]. Based on their series of patients, clinicians focused on the prognostic value of organ damage and they tended to minimise the importance of blood pressure measurement itself. In 1927, Pellissier [17] wrote "*The actual blood pressure readings themselves are not of primary importance, not even the value of the minimum pressure. As remarked by Dehon and Heitz, to claim that a patient whose minimum pressure exceeds 13 or 14 centimetres of mercury is in short-term danger of death is a gross exaggeration*".

Laubry also tempered the prognostic significance of blood pressure readings considered in isolation: "*Blood pressure readings are certainly a useful guide, provided they are correctly interpreted and not simply considered as numerical values [...]. I would like to repeat that the prognosis in hypertension is not proportional to the blood pressure readings*". Rather than rely on the blood pressure readings, it was by trying to detect organ damage that the European authors attempted to establish the prognosis of their patients. The heart was the key organ in this approach.

In the United States, Janeway drew attention to the prognostic significance of cardiac involvement because the heart was the organ most frequently damaged. Large series of autopsies provided statistical evidence that cardiac abnormalities were associated with a poor outcome, but left ventricular hypertrophy was not really viewed as a factor predictive of risk. At this stage it was simply considered to reflect the severity of hypertension and was regarded as a terminal event.

Radiology did not remain the only investigational method of enlargement for long. The electrocardiograph was invented in the early 20th century by the brilliant Dutch physiologist and physician, Einthoven. It soon proved to be an indispensable tool for cardiologists. The first commercially available apparatus was manufactured by the Cambridge Scientific Instrument Company in 1908. In 1912, 57 machines were sold worldwide. It did not take long for cardiologists to adopt the new invention and it opened up the field of rhythm disturbances as we know it today. Sokolow proposed, in terms of this new "electrical language", to quantify left ventricular hypertrophy by measuring the S and R waves in the precordial leads (the Sokolow-Lyon index is the arithmetic sum of the S and R waves in leads V1 and V5 or V6 — whichever is the greater. A sum greater than 35 mm signifies electrocardiographic left ventricular hypertrophy). With the Sokolow index, came the concept of electro-cardiographic hypertrophy.

17. Pellissier. *L'Hypertension artérielle solitaire* (Isolated arterial hypertension). Paris, 1927.

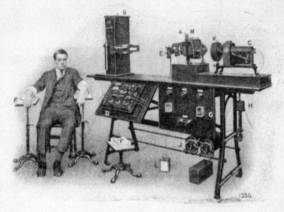

Les frais de fonctionnement de

L'Electrocardiographe
" Cambridge "

sont pratiquement négligeables.

La disposition de l'appareil est très convenable et les opérations nécessaires à l'obtention d'électrocardiogrammes satisfaisants sont extrêmement simples. En se servant du nouveau système sensible à deux fibres, on augmente beaucoup l'utilité de l'appareil. Ledit système consiste en deux fils de verre montés côte à côte dans la même boîte. On peut les régler et les employer indépendamment l'un de l'autre pour obtenir simultanément sur la même plaque des phonocardiogrammes et des électrocardiogrammes.

Nous adressons à tout demandeur la liste n° 307 qui donne tous détails de l'appareil.

THE CAMBRIDGE SCIENTIFIC Cambridge
INSTRUMENT COMPANY Ltd. Angleterre

The Electrocardiograph

The first commercially available electrocardiograph was manufactured by the Cambridge Scientific Instrument Company in 1908. In 1912, 57 machines were sold worldwide. This advertisement appeared in the French medical journal *Archives du coeur, des vaisseaux et du sang* (Archives of the heart, vessels and blood) in 1915.

The caption reads: "*The operating costs of the Cambridge Electrocardiograph are practically negligible*". The advertisement explains that: "*the arrangement of the apparatus is very convenient and the operations required to obtain a satisfactory electrocardiogram are extremely simple. By using the new sensitive two-fibre system, the usefulness of the apparatus is enhanced considerably. The system consists of two glass threads mounted side by side in the same box. They can be set and used independently to obtain simultaneously on the same plate a phonocardiogram and an electrocardiogram.*
List no. 307 provides all the details of the apparatus and can be obtained on request".

The electrocardiograph was initially used to study rhythm disturbances and was later applied to the study of ventricular hypertrophy (Sokolow), which radiological studies had already shown to be of poor prognostic significance in hypertension. In 1969, the Framingham study confirmed the prognostic validity of electrocardiographic signs of left ventricular hypertrophy.

In 1969, the Framingham study revealed that electrocardiographic evidence of left ventricular hypertrophy was a poor prognostic factor in patients, independently of their level of blood pressure [18]. Similar conclusions were reached in a large prospective study of 19,000 middle-aged men in France, published in 1989 [19].

The electrocardiographic approach encountered some methodological difficulties. Helmcke, who in 1957 studied the regression of left ventricular hypertrophy on antihypertensive treatment, expressed major reservations as to the diagnostic validity of electrocardiography [20]. Investigators in the Framingham study also drew attention to the ambiguous significance of electrocardiography which in fact reflected ischaemic phenomena, and not hypertrophy itself. The advent of echocardiography swept aside these reservations.

At the end of the 1970s, echocardiography underwent rapid expansion, bringing with it considerable qualitative and quantitative advantages over electrocardiography. From a qualitative standpoint, it became possible to measure the actual ventricular mass and not simply its electrical image. Quantitatively speaking, left ventricular hypertrophy evolved from a binary variable (present or absent) to a continuous variable measured in grams per square metre of body surface area [21].

This quantitative approach enabled a more detailed analysis of studies correlating the regression of left ventricular hypertrophy with antihypertensive therapy. By means of this new evaluation technique, Casale and Devereux confirmed for the first time in 1986 that cardiac enlargement measured by echocardiography could predict cardiovascular events in hypertensive patients after adjusting for other variables such as blood pressure levels, age or ventricular function at rest [22].

Left ventricular hypertrophy was no longer considered as a terminal event, related to the deleterious effects of hypertension on the heart, but as an independent risk factor. This did not necessarily imply a causal relationship between hypertrophy and death. Left ventricular hypertrophy may simply have been a reflection of the haemodynamic conditions to which the patient had been subjected throughout his lifetime. Viewed in this light, ventricular hypertrophy was not a risk factor (causal factor) but a marker of risk (an indirect reflection of the effects of other factors).

In over a century, the significance of left ventricular hypertrophy has thus changed radically. From an anatomical observation in cadavers (Morgagni and Bright) it became a morbid manifestation detectable by radiology and capable of predicting an unfavourable outcome in severe or long-standing hypertension, and finally it acquired the status of a risk factor identifiable by echocardiography in asymptomatic patients with moderate hypertension. Both blood pressure levels and left ventricular hypertrophy (quantified by left ventricular mass) are quantitatively correlated with risk, the higher the

18. In this study, the other factors were not subjected to a multivariate statistical analysis but to a subgroup analysis. Kannel W.B., Gordon T., Offutt D., "Left ventricular hypertrophy by electrocardiogram. Prevalence, incidence and mortality in the Framingham study". *Ann Int Med* 1969; 71: 89-101.

19. Girerd X., Darné B., Lang T. et al. Mortalité cardiovasculaire en fonction de l'hypertrophie ventriculaire gauche électrique dans une population d'hommes (Cardiovascular mortality as a function of electrocardiographic signs of left ventricular hypertrophy in a male population). *Presse méd* 1989.18: 332-335.

20. Helmcke J.G., Shneckloth R., Corcoran A.C. Electrocardiographic changes of left ventricular hypertrophy: effects of antihypertensive treatment. *Am Heart J* 1957; 553-549.

21. The validity of these measurements was established by Devereux in 1976 using comparisons with autopsy data.

22. Casale P.N., Devereux R.B. et al. Value of echocardiographic measurements of left ventricular mass in predicting cardiovascular and morbid events in hypertensive men. *Ann Int Med* 1986; n° 105 p. 173.

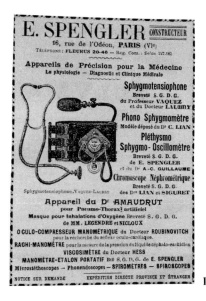

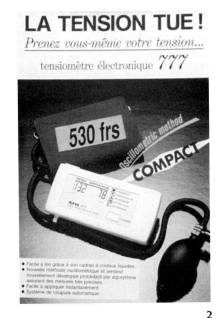

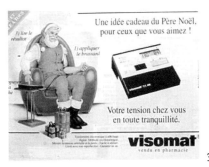

Blood pressure for sale

Sphygmomanometers were not only scientific instruments, they were also seen to have a potentially large commercial market. In 1919, Vaquez and Laubry signed a contract with the manufacturer Spengler for the production of the famous "Vaquez-Laubry Sphygmotensiophone" which was a huge commercial success in France.

Advertising, initially confined to the medical profession (*figure 1*), is now aimed at the general public who are being encouraged to take their own blood pressure.

The advertisements shown here appeared in the popular press in France in the 1990s. They appeal to the emotions of fear (Blood pressure kills ! - *figure 2*) or sentimentality (A gift for your loved ones - *figure 3*). The social dimension of blood pressure measurement will no doubt assume greater importance in the years to come.

value the higher the risk. But the relationship between the two factors is a complex one, the one being a causal factor for the other in pathophysiological terms. The elucidation of the sequence of causal events will entail studying the reversibility of risk on cessation of exposure to the risk factors analysed jointly. This will require new statistical, methodological and pathophysiological approaches, notably the assessment of the impact of pharmacologically distinct treatment [23].

From 1960 to 1990, therapeutic trials addressed the question of the level of blood pressure above which treatment provided more advantages than disadvantages for the patient. At the end of the 1980s, many studies and meta-analyses were published. Although many questions remain unanswered, the benefits and risks of treatment have now been essentially established for the various terminal events related to hypertension, including cardiac failure.

TREATMENT, PREVENTION AND PROTEST

To summarise, at the turn of the 20th century, hypertension was a symptomatic disorder for which the patients would consult their doctor who did what he could to relieve their suffering. As clinical medicine, epidemiology and pharmacology unveiled new data, prevention assumed an increasingly important role. Today in Western countries, it is even probable that individuals are more at risk of being treated inappropriately than of not being diagnosed correctly. Whereas in previous times hypertension was a dangerous malignant disease with multiple symptoms, today it has become a silent, long-term threat. In an attempt to head off the silent chronology of morbid events, doctors are performing more and more tests and "check-ups". Encouraged by the statistics, they are treating their "patients", formerly considered as normal individuals, before clinical signs appear. There is confusion between treatment and prevention. Unlike vaccination, where clearly the aim is to prevent an infection in a healthy individual, "treating" hypertension means trying to influence an uninterrupted sequence of multifactorial events leading to symptoms. The best news for a hypertensive patient is no news. Not all asymptomatic subjects will escape unharmed from this process, for which they do not always understand the need or the consequences. Voices have been raised in protest, amongst which the most boisterous (not to use the word "resounding") was that of Ivan Illich who published his best-seller *Medical Nemesis* in 1975 [24] at a time when the treatment of hypertension was being given official recognition.

In our never-ending endeavour to head off symptoms (such useful landmarks for patients), we are coming precariously close to normality to prevent the progression of cardiovascular alterations "as early as possible". The risk-benefit curve for the management of hypertension is an exponential one and there is a tendency to venture out further and further on this curve for a smaller and smaller benefit. We will not be able to continue forever with impunity.

23. Are all antihypertensive agents equivalent in reversing left ventricular hypertrophy ? The results of the Medical Research Council trial begun in 1973 and published in 1985 provides a partial answer to this question. Antihypertensive therapy was shown to reduce the incidence of elctrocardiographic signs of left ventricular hypertrophy. This effect was more pronounced with the thiazide diuretics than with betablockers, after adjusting for blood pressure levels. The authors suggested that the thiazides may prevent hypertrophy via a metabolic mechanism.
In: *Mild hypertension - is there pressure to treat?* Miall W.E., Greenberg G., on behalf of the MRC's working party. Cambridge University Press, Cambridge. 1987 pp. 82-83.
A more ambitious and crucial question faces investigators in the 1990s: does the regression of left ventricular hypertrophy, obtained by antihypertensive treatment, reduce morbidity and mortality independently of the lowering of blood pressure? The question remains open.

24. Ivan Illich, philosopher, theologist and sociologist published a frankly anti-medical book in 1975 entitled *Medical Nemesis* (Calder and Boyers Publ. London. 1975) in which he states that: *"The medical establishment may be hazardous to your health"*. On hypertension he writes: *" The drug treatment of high blood pressure is effective and warrants the risk of side-effects in the few in whom it is a malignant condition; it represents a considerable risk of serious harm, far outweighing any proven benefit, for the 10 to 20 million Americans on whom rash artery-plumbers are trying to foist it"*.

8
THE GENETICS OF ARTERIAL HYPERTENSION

Diseases sometimes have a family destiny, as Royal families with haemophilia are well aware. Since ancient times, cattle breeders have known that they could perpetuate desirable characteristics from one generation to the next, and very early on, physicians turned their attention to the question of heredity[1]. Well before the era of genetics, the concept of "diathesis" was very popular and supported the idea of a predisposition to disease, a sort of "morbid susceptibility" that individuals exhibited to gout, tuberculosis, or asthma for example. In 1876, before blood pressure began to be measured, Dieulafoy called attention to the *"considerable role that heredity appears to play in the production of cerebral haemorrhage"*[2]. Closer to modern times, in 1923, Rosenbloom reported a family of hypertensive individuals and remarked that *"if it is true that we know today that some diseases are hereditary, it is not generally known that there is a hereditary type of hypertension"*[3]. Two years later, Ayman published a study showing that there was a high incidence of hypertension amongst family members of patients hospitalised for hypertension and he concluded that *"heredity is the most important factor in the development of essential hypertension"*. His impression was confirmed by the observation of a Jewish family which had recently emigrated from Russia to Boston and in which hypertension was found in members of three generations[4]. In 1934, the same author published a study involving 1,524 members of 277 families[5]. The great adventure of the genetics of hypertension was about to begin.

HISTORICAL BIOMETRIC STUDIES IN FAMILIES AND TWINS

In the 1970s, family studies and studies in mono or dizygotic twins established that blood pressure was in part transmitted genetically. These studies also quantified the relative contribution of genetic factors. It was thus shown that there was a correlation between the blood pressure of parents and children. But very quickly it became apparent that the environment also played an important role in the level of blood pressure, with a more marked influence in adults. A certain degree of similarity was also demonstrated in the blood pressure of spouses, related essentially to their similarity for weight. Studies performed in monozygotic twins

1. For the history of heredity, see: François Jacob. *La logique du vivant* (The logic of the living). 1970. Gallimard, Paris.

2. Dieulafoy M. Rôle de l'hérédité dans la production de l'hémorragie cérébrale (The role of heredity in the production of cerebral haemorrhage). *Gazette Hebdo Med Chir* 1876; 38: 595-597.

3. Rosenbloom J., Pittsburgh Ph.D. Familial hypertension with report of a case. *J Lab Clin Med* 1923; 8: 681-693.

4. Ayman D. The hereditary aspect of arteriolar (essential) hypertension. *N Engl J Med* 1933, July 27th, pp. 194-197.

5. Ayman D. Heredity in arteriolar (essential) hypertension. *Arch Intern Med* 1934, 53: 792-802.

whose genetic make-up is identical provided a means for quantifying the influence of the environment and of genetic factors on observed differences in blood pressure. One of the most elegant studies designed to evaluate the respective roles of genetics and the environment in the determination of blood pressure was performed in 1976 by Annest et al. in French Canadian families with both natural and adopted children [6]. The natural and adopted children shared the same environment and it was therefore possible to differenciate between the influence of purely hereditary factors and that of common environmental factors. This study showed that there was a stronger correlation between the blood pressures of natural siblings than between those of adopted siblings.

This inter-individual variability, evaluated on the basis of quantitative genetic methods, is composed of a genetic variance (ranging from 20% to 50% in different studies with a generally accepted value of 30%) and environmental, non-genetic variance (of the order of 50%). It must be recognised, however, that these figures are subject to a substantial margin of inaccuracy and that they only apply to the populations studied in Western societies (there is no comparable data for developing countries). Furthermore, these "historic" data will be difficult to reproduce because today families tend to be scattered and hypertension is rapidly treated so that collecting data on spontaneous blood pressure levels in hypertensive individuals becomes arduous.

ONE OR SEVERAL GENES RESPONSIBLE FOR HYPERTENSION ? THE PICKERING-PLATT CONTROVERSY

A hereditary disease may simply be associated with a single gene (monogenic disease), usually with a mendelian mode of transmission. In such cases, it is relatively easy to identify the gene responsible using current techniques of molecular genetics. Other diseases on the contrary result from abnormalities of more than one gene (oligogenic) or even multiple genes (polygenic). In these cases, the mode of transmission is more complex and not mendelian. Over 30 years ago, George Pickering and Robert Platt debated this problem. Their arguments were based on the analysis of blood pressure distribution curves in different populations. The bimodal distribution of blood pressure noted by Platt led him to separate quite clearly a normotensive population and a hypertensive population. He concluded that hypertension was therefore a hereditary disease associated with a single morbid gene. In contrast, Pickering found a unimodal distribution for both systolic and diastolic blood pressure with no distinct discrimination between normotensive and hypertensive individuals [7]. He therefore proposed that hypertension was a polygenic disease and was not the result of a single gene defect. Today, the debate appears to be over in so far as the distribution of blood pressure in the different populations studied does indeed appear to be unimodal, even if here and there a few rare reports continue to describe a bimodal distribution. These data are consistent with findings in genetically

6. Annest J.L., Sing C.F., Biron P., Mongeau J.P. Familial aggregation of blood pressure and weight in adoptive families. *Am J Epidemiol* 1979; 110: 479-491.

7. Carnussi A., Bianchi G. Genetics of essential hypertension. From the unimodal-bimodal controversy to molecular technology. *Hypertension* 1988; 12: 620-628.

hypertensive animals. In the genetically hypertensive Dahl rat, fed a high salt diet, it appears that at least 4 to 6 genes are responsible for the elevation of blood pressure. Today, there is general agreement that blood pressure is dependent on multiple genetic and environmental factors.

THE SEARCH FOR THE CAUSAL GENES: INITIAL APPROACH BY THE STUDY OF INTERMEDIATE PHENOTYPES

Blood pressure is dependent on several genes and their products. The genes do not act directly on the phenotypic trait i.e. blood pressure, but rather through a relay mechanism which amplifies and modulates their message. The actions of the genes are thus transmitted through a whole series of physiological events. This idea of a phenotype close to the gene (enzyme, receptor, growth factor...) and intermediate phenotype (cell and tissue function...) and distal phenotype (the level of blood pressure) was popularised by R.R. Williams [8]. In fact, the level of blood pressure is the result of the integration of a considerable number of biological events. The "intermediate phenotype" is composed of all the measurable variables, the indicators of the expression of the genes from the cell level to clinical arterial pressure. To be incriminated in the determination of familial hypertension, these intermediate phenotypes must satisfy two criteria. First, there must be a relationship between the level of blood pressure and the variations of the intermediate phenotype under consideration and second, familial aggregation of the phenotype must be shown.

The most well-studied intermediate phenotype is that of ion flux in blood cells, particularly the increase of sodium-lithium exchange in red blood cells. This is the best characterised sodium transport abnormality in hypertensive individuals. These studies had the advantage of providing a relatively simple test and their results raised hopes that the abnormalities detected in the erythrocytes would also be found in vascular smooth muscle cells of hypertensive patients. About 15 years ago, it was shown that increased sodium-lithium counter-transport could precede the onset of hypertension and that it may represent a biological marker of hypertension [9]. The analysis of the distribution of sodium-lithium exchange revealed the presence of a bimodal curve suggesting that a variable form of what was probably a single gene was responsible for the high level of counter-transport. However, the level of counter-transport plays only a relatively minor role in the overall level of blood pressure (3 to 5 mmHg). Many other intermediate phenotypes have been studied in human hypertension, such as plasma angiotensinogen, and angiotensin I converting enzyme, urinary kallicrein, salt sensitivity and the response to pharmacological agents. The analysis of the results obtained gave rise to hypotheses on the effect of the alleles, dominant or not, but the gene responsible for the quantitative differences in expression and the alleles involved in variable levels of expression remained to be identified. This has now become possible through molecular genetics.

8. Williams R.R., Hunt S.C., Hasstedt S.J., Berry T.D., Wu L.L., Barlow G.K., Stults B.M., Kuida H. Definition of genetic factors in hypertension: a search for major genes, polygenes, and homogeneous subtypes. *J Cardiovasc Pharmacol* 1988; 12 (suppl)): S7-S20.

9. Canessa M., Adragna N., Solomon S., Conolly T.N., Tosteson D.C. Increased sodium-lithium counter-transport in red cells of patients with essential hypertension. *N Engl J Med* 1980; 302: 722-726.

NEW ADVANCES IN HYPERTENSION
THROUGH MOLECULAR GENETICS

Molecular genetics has provided a new approach to the pathophysiology of hypertension through the study of genetic polymorphism. Variations in DNA sequence can be detected by molecular biology techniques, thus enabling a specific genotype to be defined for each individual. The remarkable progress of molecular genetics over the past 10 years means that it is now possible to envision the identification of the genes responsible for variations in blood pressure and, within these genes themselves, to pinpoint the regions which may play a determinant role in hypertension. Spectacular results have been achieved in the rare monogenic forms of early and severe hypertension. It will be far more difficult to identify the genes responsible for more common forms of essential hypertension in man.

MONOGENIC FORMS OF HYPERTENSION

Monogenic forms of hypertension usually have an early and severe onset. They were described and characterised by paediatricians almost 30 years ago, but it was only after 1992 that three monogenic forms of hypertension were identified genetically. In 1992, the gene responsible for one of these forms, dexamethasone-sensitive hypertension was identified for the first time [10]. Transmitted as an autosomal dominant trait, this form of hypertension is accompanied by a decrease in serum potassium and renin, and an increased secretion of aldosterone. It is cured by the administration of glucocorticoids (dexamethasone). The abnormality is related to a supernumerary chimaeric gene resulting from the fusion of two genes coding for the enzymes involved in aldosterone biosynthesis.

10. Lifton R.P., Dluhy R.G., Powers M., Rich G.M., Cook S., Ulick S., Lalouel J.M. A chimaeric 11ß-hydroxylase/aldosterone synthase gene causes glucocorticoid-remediable aldosteronism and hypertension. *Nature* 1992; 355: 262-265.

The syndrome of apparent excess of mineralocorticoid secretion is a recessive disorder resulting from the inactivation of an enzyme which breaks down cortisol. The latter accumulates in the distal tubular cells of the kidney where aldosterone exerts its effect and illegitimately occupies the mineralocorticoid receptor. Finally, a syndrome described in 1963 by Liddle (called Liddle's syndrome) has recently found a molecular explanation. Patients suffering from this autosomal dominant disorder present with severe hypertension and decreased levels of renin and aldosterone. Liddle observed that patients could be cured by the administration of triamterene or amiloride, diuretics which act on the renal cells which are the targets for aldosterone. Amiloride blocks a sodium channel activated by aldosterone. Liddle's hypothesis was that a constitutional activation of this channel induced reabsorption of sodium. This hypothesis was confirmed in 1994 by the discovery of a mutation in one of the chains composing this channel in several families suffering from the syndrome. These discoveries are good illustrations of how the progress of the molecular genetics of monogenic diseases has been applied to the study of hypertension.

The discovery of specific genetic defects underlying certain cases of hypertension has raised hopes that the more common forms of "essential" hypertension may also find an explanation in the mechanisms thus uncovered. The three forms of monogenic hypertension described above are characterised by an abnormally high rate of reabsorption of sodium and water and an expansion of extra-cellular fluid. They are enhanced by salt intake and thus resemble forms of essential hypertension in which increased salt sensitivity has been found and appears to be genetically determined. One of the current hypotheses is that certain forms of essential hypertension with increased salt sensitivity could have as their basis an abnormality of one of the genes responsible for the three identified forms of monogenic hypertension. Another interesting observation is the variable effect of the chimaeric gene responsible for dexamethasone-sensitive hypertension. According to recent family studies, the effect of this gene results in a rise in blood pressure of approximately 30 mmHg. This is a mean effect however because certain families exhibiting the genetic abnormality do not have an abnormal elevation of their blood pressure. In such cases, it may be that the non-affected family member has a particularly low level of blood pressure, a trait which could also be genetically determined. Results like these again suggest that blood pressure might be viewed as a quantitative trait resulting from the algebraic sum of "morbid hypertensive" genes and "protective anti-hypertensive" genes.

NEW STRATEGIES: EXPERIMENTAL APPROACHES

The ability to produce genetically determined hypertension in laboratory animals paved the way for an experimental approach to the problem. At the end of the 1950s, Smirk and his coworkers succeeded in creating a strain of genetically hypertensive rats by cross-breeding rats with spontaneously elevated blood pressure [11]. By cross-breeding several generations, they ended up with a genetically hypertensive strain of rat. The same procedure was used to develop other models of genetically hypertensive rats (Japanese SHR rats, Lyons rats, Milan strain, etc.). In these strains of rats, the inheritance of high blood pressure may affect 60% of the animals. One advantage of using such pure strains is that it enables the study of a single group of genes causing hypertension. Another advantage is that they can be used to identify and control environmental factors which are superimposed on the genetic factors in determining blood pressure. It is possible to identify genetic polymorphisms between the strains of rats used in the cross-breeding of hypertensive and normotensive animals, and to look for cosegregation of these markers with blood pressure in the offspring. Rapp and his co-workers were the first to identify a locus involved in hypertension by using a genetic marker on the renin gene [12]. They showed that salt-sensitive Dahl rats had hypertension which cosegregates with a marker

11. Smirk F.H., Hall W.H. Inherited hypertension in rats. *Nature* 1958; 182: 727.

12. Rapp J.H., Wang S.M., Dene H. A genetic polymorphism in the renin gene of Dahl rats cosegregates with blood pressure. *Science* 1989; 243: 542-544.

on the renin gene. This genetic linkage indicates that the renin gene, or a gene close to it, is responsible for the elevation of blood pressure. The genetic marker used, in this case the renin gene, is an illustration of the so-called "candidate gene" approach.

Another approach consists of looking for a locus which cosegregates with blood pressure by using polymorphic markers distributed throughout the rat genome. By using this "positional cloning" technique, Marc Lathrop's group [13] and Eric Lander's group [14], working with the offspring of interbred normotensive and hypertensive rats, achieved a breakthrough in the field of polygenic disorders. They identified two main loci, one of which contained the gene coding for the angiotensin converting enzyme. It remains to be determined which gene or genes within these loci are responsible for the elevation of blood pressure under basal conditions or after salt overloading. This inverse genetic approach has been used successfully in the study of monogenic diseases and it should also find an application in oligogenic or polygenic disorders.

MOLECULAR GENETICS OF HUMAN ESSENTIAL HYPERTENSION: THE FIRST STEP

The molecular genetics of human essential hypertension is a recent development made possible by the emergence of molecular genetic techniques applied to polygenic diseases. The candidate gene approach described above in animal models has so far been the only one used. The aim here is to demonstrate an elementary vertical relationship between these candidate genes, the intermediate phenotypes and their effects on blood pressure. As more and more relationships of this type are reported, it will become possible to assign an effect on blood pressure to a specific allele. In the example of the renin system, the vertical relationship consists of recognising the alleles of the different genes, measuring their effects on the activity of this system in patients and determining their influence on the level of blood pressure. This approach exemplifies one of the ways in which medical reasoning works. Probably the best example of this approach today is the discovery of the possible role of angiotensinogen in the determination of essential hypertension. Jeunemaître and his coworkers [15] demonstrated a relationship between the angiotensinogen gene and blood pressure in pairs of siblings with hypertension and they discovered a variant of angiotensinogen more commonly observed in hypertensive than in normotensive individuals.

Finally, they showed that this variant in the homozygous state was associated with an elevation of plasma angiotensinogen of the order of 20%. And so, the linear relationship is complete between a gene variant (the angiotensinogen gene), and intermittent phenotype (plasma level of angiotensinogen) and a distal phenotype (blood pressure). This strategy considers that hypertension is the consequence of the malfunction of a

13. Hilbert P., Lindpaintner K., Beckmann J., Serikawa T., Soubrier F., Dubay C., Cartwright P., De Gouyon B., Julier C., Takahashi S., Vincent M., Ganten D., Georges M., Lathrop M. Chromosomal mapping of two genetic loci associated with blood pressure regulation in hereditary hypertensive rats. *Nature* 1991; 353: 521-526.

14. Jacob H.L., Lindpaintner K., Lincoln S.E., Kusumi K., Bunker R.K., Mao Y.P., Ganten D., Dzau V.J. Lander E.S. Genetic mapping of a gene causing hypertension in the stroke-prone spontaneously hypertensive rat. *Cell* 1991; 67: 213-224.

15. Jeunemaître X., Soubrier F., Kotelevtsev Y., Lifton R., Williams C.S., Charru A., Hunt S.C. Hopkins P.N., Williams R.R., Lalouel J.M., Corvol P. Molecular basis of human hypertension: role of angiotensinogen. *Cell* 1992; 71:169-180.

limited number of well-identified regulatory systems and it attempts to analyse them one by one at the genetic level. A totally different approach is to concentrate on genetic linkages within families or pairs of siblings, a valuable source of information because of the number of affected individuals, the severity of the trait or the special features that the disease may exhibit. As in the rat, the aim here is to look for a genetic linkage between the disease and markers throughout the genome. This requires collecting clinical and biological data from large families of hypertensive individuals, immortalising lymphocytes, and major computer facilities for analysing the data. Having identified a linkage with a given locus, the aim then is to identify the gene responsible within that locus.

Clearly this is difficult research, but the stakes are high. What patients want to know is what is their risk of developing hypertension and what should they do about it in terms of lifestyle modifications. They also want to understand the reasons for being treated. To answer these haunting questions, the physician has to be able to evaluate the patient's genetic predisposition to cardiovascular disease in general, and to hypertension in particular. This means identifying the genes that render an individual sensitive to a given factor in the environment.

EPILOGUE

The future?

A century has elapsed since blood presure was first measured non-invasively in man. During those one hundred years, medicine has undergone profound changes, driven by the progress in biology and the exact sciences. From the emergence of the concept of risk through to the promise of effective therapy, hypertension has followed, but also to some extent contributed actively to this evolution. We have come a long way. Admittedly there is still room for improvement: better methodology, individually-tailored treatments, improved forecasting of prognosis, pharmacological advances and so on. But who would venture to predict which of these will be the centre of attention in the coming years ?

From a scientific standpoint we can predict that in the near future, technology will modify methods used for measuring blood pressure, provide more detailed laboratory tests and advance our understanding of blood pressure regulation. In the more distant future, the genetic approach to hypertension might revolutionise both the way we view hypertension and the way we treat it. One can try to predict the future of hypertension by gazing into the crystal ball of biomedical research, but one must remember that each technological step forward will have its consequences on how the hypertensive patient is managed.

The debate over threshold levels will continue to evolve. No doubt, therapeutic strategies will be more directed to tailoring treatment to the individual patient and we will begin to think in terms of "target pressure" rather than threshold levels. The scientific future of cardiovascular disorders will also be subject to unpredictable socio-cultural and economic influences. In 1996, we cannot foresee the impact of the economic restrictions which are likely to conflict with a purely scientific logic. But to what extent ? Medical ethics are bound to change and already the word "patient" is being replaced by the term "subject examined". The future of hypertension thus shares a common destiny with science, economics and the cultural choices we make for our society. It seems only fitting to let Gallavardin have the final word: *From all that has been said, and taking into account the large number of factors that can modify blood pressure, in either direction, we may conclude that the physician who sets out to follow the variations in blood pressure has a particularly ardous task ahead of him and that this undertaking is based on very unstable foundations*".

MILESTONES

1628 • Discovery of blood circulation by William Harvey.

1661 • Publication of the first bills of mortality in England by John Graunt.

1679 • Theoretical calculation of the "*force of the heart*" by Borelli.

1733 • First experimental measurement of blood pressure by Stephen Hales.

1749 • Sénac indicates that the volume of the heart can increase and reflects on "the force of the dilated heart".

1778 • First mortality tables produced by a life insurance company in England.

1819 • Laënnec invents the stethoscope and inaugurates the anatomico-clinical approach with the Paris School of Medicine.

1824 • The Clerical Medical and General insurance company sets up a medical department.

1828 • Invention of the haemodynamometer by Poiseuille who publishes a thesis on *The force of the blood*.

1831 • Use of the word "*pressure*" by Richard Bright (but with a meaning different from arterial pressure).

1832 • Pierre Charles Alexandre Louis (founder of the numerate method) sets up the *Medical Observation Society*.

1834 • Invention of the sphygmometer by Hérisson to "*provide a visual reflection of the action of the arteries*".

1836 • Richard Bright reports that most patients who die of renal failure have left ventricular hypertrophy at autopsy.

1847 • Ludwig's kymograph.

1854 • Karl von Vierodt's sphygmograph.

1856 • Direct intra-arterial measurement of blood pressure in man during an amputation by the surgeon Faivre.

1860 • Jules-Etienne Marey presents his sphygmograph to the Academy of Medicine.

1865 • Use of the term "*milieu intérieur*" by Claude Bernard.

1870 • Use of the clinical thermometer to measure body temperature by Thomas Clifford Allbutt.

1871 • Ludwig Traube in Germany suggests a link between renal failure and elevated blood pressure due to renal obstruction.

1872 • William Gull and Gawen Sutton in England accuse the systemic capillary system of causing left ventricular hypertrophy in patients with renal failure.

1874 • In North America, 200 life insurance companies had already sold over one million policies.

1876 • The role of heredity in certain cases of cerebral haemorrhage suggested by Dieulafoy.

• Gowers studies the state of the arteries in Bright's disease using the ophthalmoscope.

1881 • Victor Basch in Germany describes the first sphygmomanometer able to measure blood pressure non-invasively in humans.

1887 • Nitrate derivates recommended as hypotensive agents by Huchard.

1889 • Brown-Séquard quotes the kidney as an example of an internally secreting organ.

• Potain's sphygmomanometer.

1894 • Oliver and Schäfer show that adrenal extracts can raise blood pressure.

1895 • Discovery of x-rays by Röntgen.

1896 • Riva-Rocci presents his inflatable cuff at the Italian Congress of Internal Medicine and publishes his invention in the *Gazzetta Medica di Torino*.

• In Italy, Mosso invents an instrument to measure blood pressure at the extremity of the fingers.

1896 • d'Arsonval in France reports having lowered the blood pressure of a dog by electrotherapy.

1898 • Tigerstedt and Bergman show blood pressure elevation in rabbits after injection of a renal extract which they call "*renin*".

1899 • Gaertner invents the "*tonometer*" with a pneumatic ring placed on the second phalanx of the finger.

• First sympathectomy for arterial disease by the French surgeon Jaboulay.

1901 • Isolation of adrenaline by Jokichi Takamine.

1902 • Posthumous publication of Potain's book *Human blood pressure in health and disease*.

1903 • Wolfgang Pauli describes the hypotensive effects of sodium nitroprussate.

• Electrotherapy used for the first time in man to lower blood pressure.

1904 • Synthesis of adrenaline by Stolz.

• Ambard and Beaujard show that "*chloride unloading*" can lower blood pressure in patients with Bright's disease.

1905 • Nicolaï Korotkoff describes an auscultatory method for measuring blood pressure.

1908 • The first electrocardiograph become available.

• First issue of the journal *Archives des maladies du coeur, des vaisseaux et du sang* (Archives of the heart, vessels and blood), the first French journal of cardiology and haematology.

1909 • First issue of *Heart*, the first English language journal of cardiology.

1911 • Fischer, medical director of the Northwestern Mutual Life Company recommends measuring blood pressure in all life insurance applicants.

1913 • Theodore Janeway in the United States publishes his first series of hypertensive patients from among his private patients.

1913 • Vaquez recommends the use of radioscopy to monitor heart size in patients with Bright's disease and suggests that radioscopic evidence of left ventricular hypertrophy can reveal hypertension.

• Leriche shows that sympathetic denervation induces vasodilatation and increases blood flow in the corresponding territory.

• Cottenot publishes his thesis on irradiation of the adrenals in hypertension.

1914 • Volhard and Fahr describe the clinical picture of malignant hypertension.

• Life insurance companies show a statistical relationship between abdominal circumference and life expectancy.

1915 • The Prudential Life Insurance company publishes statistics based on the blood pressure of 18,637 applicants.

• Allbutt in the United States proposes the term "*hyperpiesia*" for high blood pressure of unknown cause.

• The relationship between alcohol consumption and hypertension is established by Lian.

1916 • A French publication claims that the blood pressure of soldiers in the trenches reflects objectively the state of fatigue of a battalion.

1917 • "*The higher the arterial tension, the greater the mortality*", writes Fischer in the proceedings of the Association of Life Insurance Medical Directors of America.

1919 • Vaquez and Laubry conceive a sphygmomanometer manufactured and sold by Spengler.

1920 • Louis Gallavardin publishes the second edition of his book *Blood pressure in clinical medicine*.

1921 • Henri Vaquez criticises French life insurance companies for not measuring blood pressure routinely.

1922
- Labbé publishes a case of paroxysmal hypertension with an adrenal tumour.
- Discovery of insulin.

1923
- Rosenbloom reports a family of hypertensives.

1925
- Rowntree and Addison in the United States perform the first lumbar sympathectomy for malignant hypertension.

1927
- Charles Mayo performs the first resection of a pheochromocytoma without knowing what he was resecting.

1929
- Pincoffs operates on a patient with a preoperative diagnosis of pheochromocytoma.
- The medical impairment study by life insurance companies, shows a relationship between obesity and blood pressure.

1930 (approx)
- Mortality due to degenerative diseases overtakes mortality due to infectious diseases. This is the beginning of the "epidemiological transition".

1931
- In an editorial, Riesman interprets essential hypertension as a disease due to "the American way of life".
- Rauwolfia serpentina, a new Indian drug, is shown to be effective in hypertension.

1933
- Reserpine, an alkaloid from Rauwolfia serpentina is shown to lower blood pressure.

1934
- First successful experimental model of hypertension by Harry Goldblatt.
- Ayman publishes a series of 1,524 hypertensive patients from 277 families.

1939
- The Blood Pressure Study combines statistics from 15 North American insurance companies and totals 1,309,000 insurance policy holders.
- Keith and Wagener propose using a 4-category classification for more reliable study of the evolution and prognosis of hypertension.

1940
- Braun-Menéndez and Page propose the term angiotensin.
- Smithwick describes his technique of lumber splanchnicectomy.
- Ayman proposes using blood pressure measurement taken at home (by the patient or his family).

1942
- Penicillin becomes commercially available.

1944
- Kempner's "rice diet".

1946
- Pentaquine becomes the first orally active agent in malignant hypertension.

1947
- Start of the Framingham study.
- Peet refines the indications for splanchnicectomy.

1948
- Kempner publishes the results of the dietary treatment (protein diet) of 500 hypertensive patients.
- Alquist proposes a classification of adrenergic receptors.

1949
- Creation of the National Heart Institute
- Pyrotherapy used in malignant hypertension.
- Sokolow and Lyon propose an index to quantify electrocardiographic left ventricular hypertrophy.

1950
- Hexamethonium, first antihypertensive ganglion blocker, becomes commercially available.

1952
- Isolation of aldosterone and synthesis of cortisone.

1953
- Introduction of hydralazine.
- Watson and Crick describe the molecular structure of DNA.

1954
- Steggs et al. in the U.S.A. and Peart et al. in the U.K. isolate and determine the sequence of angiotensin I and II.

1954 • First clinical use of echocardiography.

1955 • Conn describes primary aldosteronism on the basis of a single clinical case.

1956 • Synthesis of reserpine.

1957 • First clinical results with chlorothiazide reported by Freis at the American Heart Congress.

1958 • Synthesis of Angiotensin II by Schwyer and coworkers.

• Publication of the results of medical treatment for malignant hypertension by Dustin and Page.

1959 • Report of hypotensive effects of bretylium and guanethidine.

• Hydrochlorothiazide becomes available.

1960 • First ambulatory recordings of blood pressure by Sokolow.

1961 • Continuous recording of the electro-cardiogram by Holter.

1962 • First continuous recording of blood pressure by a direct intra-arterial method.

• Introduction of verapamil as a smooth muscle relaxant.

• First clinical trials of pronethalol by James Black.

1963 • Start of the Veterans Administration trial in hypertension to test hydrochloro-thiazide, reserpine or hydralazine against placebo.

• Fleckenstein studies the mechanism of action of verapamil, considered to be a betablocker.

1964 • Propanolol becomes available for the treatment of angina pectoris and publications suggest it is effective in hypertension.

1965 • Ferreira isolates from snake poison a substance which potentiates the effects of bradykinin.

1966 • Discovery of nifedipine.

• Clonidine used in everyday medical practice.

1967 • The Veterans Administration study directed by Freis establishes the benefits of treating moderate hypertension in a randomised, placebo-controlled trial.

1969 • Fleckenstein suggests a new pharma-cological class — the calcium channel blockers.

• The Framingham study demonstrates a statistical relationship between electro-cardiographic ventricular hypertrophy and prognosis.

1971 • Report of the first angiotensin converting enzyme inhibitor.

1976 • Annest publishes a study on the influence of genetics and the environment on blood pressure in natural and adopted siblings.

1978 • First clinical trials of captopril.

1982 • Beta-blockers belatedly receive FDA approval for use in hypertension.

1986 • Demonstration of the prognostic value of cardiac enlargement measured by electrocardiography.

1992 • Identification of the gene responsible for dexamethasone-sensitive hypertension.

• Demonstration of a link between the angiotensin gene and blood pressure in hypertensive siblings.

1994 • Kaplan reveals that 30% of all Americans from 55 to 64 years of age are on an antihypertensive drug (and 40% from 65 to 74).

BIOGRAPHIES

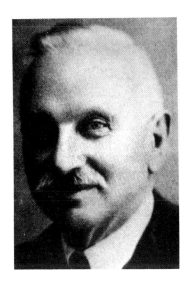

Scipione Riva-Rocci (1863-1937)

Scipione Riva-Rocci was born in Almese, a small town in the Turin province, in 1863. He graduated in medicine from the University of Turin in 1888 and then worked as assistant professor in the Institute of Clinica Medica directed by Professor Forlanini, first in the University of Turin (1888-1898) and then in the University of Pavia (1898-1900). In 1900 he became Head of the Division of Internal Medicine at the Varese Hospital where he served in the following decades. In this position he maintained a close connection with the Pavia University where he regularly taught paediatrics to the sixth-year medical students. He retired in 1928 and thereafter lived first in Milan and then in Rapallo where he died in 1937, at the age of 74.

In his years with Professor Forlanini Doctor Riva-Rocci performed much important research and was a key person in the development of the "artificial pneumothorax" which marked an important step in the treatment of pulmonary tuberculosis.

The work on blood pressure measurement, for which he later became famous, was presented in the scientific session of the Reale Accademia di Medicina di Torino on November 27th, 1896 under the title of *Un nuovo sfigmomanometro* (a new sphygmomanometer). The Riva-Rocci sphygmomanometer was then used on a limited scale for a number of experimental projects until 1901 when an American surgeon, Doctor Harvey Cushing, heard about it and visited Riva-Rocci in Pavia. Cushing thought that the Riva-Rocci sphygmomanometer was exactly what was needed to reduce intra and perioperative mortality in brain surgery. . He took it back with him to the USA and became the most enthusiastic and active supporter of the Riva-Rocci sphygmomanometer around the world. It is thus to a pioneer of neurosurgery that we owe the knowledge and use of an instrument which has been so critical for the progress of cardiovascular medicine.

Nicolai Sergeivich Korotkoff
(1874-1920)

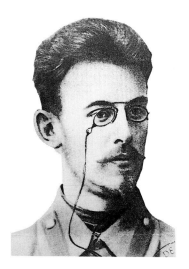

Nicolai Sergeivich Korotkoff was born on February 13th, 1874. He entered the medical faculty of Kharkov University in 1893 and transferred to Moscow University in 1895, where he graduated with distinction in 1898 at the age of twenty-four [1].

Korotkoff was given leave of absence to serve with the Russian military forces in the Far East during the Boxer Rebellion in China in 1900. He was attached to the Red Cross in the Iversh Community. The journey to the Far East entailed extensive travel by way of the Trans-Siberian railroad, through Irkutsh across Lake Baikal to Vladivostock, and he returned to Moscow via Japan, Singapore, Ceylon, and the Suez Canal to reach the Black Sea and Foedosia. He was honoured with the Order of St. Anna for "outstanding zealous labours in helping the sick and wounded soldiers" [2].

On his return Korotkoff turned his mind from military to academic pursuits and translated Albert's monograph Dir Chirurgische Diagnostik from German to Russian. In 1903, Dr. Serge P. Federov, an older colleague, was appointed professor of surgery at the Military Medical Academy at St. Petersburg, and he invited Korotkoff to join him as assistant surgeon. In the same year, Kortkoff took the first of several examinations for a doctorate of medicine.

It was not long, however, before war again interrupted his studies. During the Russo-Japanese War of 1904-5, he went to Harbin in Manchuria as senior surgeon in charge of the Second St. George's Unit of the Red Cross. He became interested in vascular surgery and began to collect cases for his doctoral thesis, which was to include 41 reports of patients he had treated during his stay in Harbin.

Returning to St. Petersburg in April 1905 he began to prepare his thesis, but it was a presentation to the Imperial Military Academy in 1905 that earned him lasting fame; the technique of blood pressure measurement was reported in less than a page of the Reports of the Imperial Military Medical Academy of St. Petersburg [3].

The critical comments of Korotkoff's peers were dealt with in an adroit manner, and he appeared a month later at the Imperial Military Academy with animal experiments to support his theory that the sounds he had

1. Laher M., O'Brien E. In search of Korotkoff. *BMJ* 1982; 285: 1796-1798.

2. Neliobova L.S. The life and scientific achievement of Dr N. S. Korotkoff. Proceedings of XLV scientific conference of the medical and pharmaceutical faculties. Kursk: 1971.

3. See chapter 1 p 6.

described were produced locally rather than in the heart [1]. He earned the approbation of Professor M. V. Yanovski, who declared: "Korotkoff has noticed and intelligently utilised a phenomenon which many observers have overlooked". These two brief communications are of greater interest to us than his thesis, which he successfully defended in 1910 [1]. Although he does refer to his technique of blood pressure measurement in the thesis, he does not describe it in any detail. In fact, were it not for Yanovski who saw the potential value of Korotkoff's technique, the auscultatory method of blood pressure measurement might have languished in obscurity. He and his pupils verified the accuracy of Korotkoff's observations and described the phases of the auscultatory sounds and for a time the technique was known as the Korotkoff-Yanovski method [1].

These three communications appear to be the sum of Korotkoff's contribution to scientific publications. The reasons as to why his academic career was not more productive have been addressed previously. In 1908 we find him serving as a research physician to the mining district Vitimsko-Olekminsky in Siberia. After receiving his doctorate he served as surgeon to the workers of the gold mines of Lensk. Here he witnessed some Tsarist atrocities, and was affected deeply by the murder of unarmed striking miners. After this he returned to St. Petersburg and during the first World War, he was surgeon to "The Charitable House for Disabled Soldiers" in Tsarskoe Selo. He welcomed the October Revolution after which he was physician-in-chief of the Metchnikov Hospital in Leningrad until his death in 1920 at the young age of 46. His wife outlived him by twenty years and died in the siege of Leningrad in December 1941 [4].

4. Segal H.N. *Experiments for determining the efficacy of arterial collaterals* by N.C. Korotkoff. Montreal: Mansfield Book Mart, 1980. (Preface biographical notes and editing of translation from Russian).

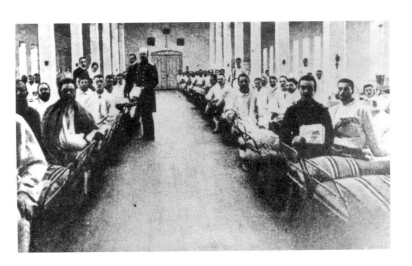

Interior of the second Hospital of the St George Red Cross Society in 1904.

Theodore Janeway (1872-1917)

Theodore Caldwell Janeway contributed much to the literature on hypertension [1-14]. His greatest work was *The Clinical Study of Blood Pressure. A guide to the Use of the Sphygmomanometer in Medical, Surgical, and Obstetrical Practice, with a Summary of the Experimental and Clinical Facts Relating to the Blood-Pressure in Health and in Disease*, which was published in 1904 [15]. A century ago Janeway was as fully aware of the sources of error in the blood pressure measuring technique to which we so frequently draw attention today, namely, the importance of ensuring that the arm is both relaxed and at heart level during measurement, that the cuff is deflated slowly, that an interval is allowed between measurements, and that *"an armlet of 12 cm width is adequate for any but the most enormous arms"* [15]. Janeway also anticipated the expansion of clinical sphygmomanometry and he recognised that this development would bring its own problems: *"The gradual development of various sphygmomanometers from which one may choose a clinical instrument today (1904), has been unfortunate in breeding more partisan bias and personal feeling than should find a place in the quest of scientific accuracy; but this evil has not been without its good side. It has led to the rigid scrutiny of each new instrument brought forward, and a diligent search for its faults"* [15]. He advocated the Riva-Rocci mercury manometer rather than the aneroid device of Hill and Barnard because the gauge became inaccurate with use and frequent recalibration was necessary, an occurrence which led Janeway to draw attention to a difficulty with which we are all too familiar with today: *"The manometer is also difficult of repair in this country, a considerable drawback to so costly an apparatus (US$40)"* [15]. To overcome this weakness, attention was directed to determining diastolic blood pressure by observing the oscillations in a mercury manometer rather than an an aneroid gauge and Janeway produced a sphygmomanometer incorporating for the first time most of the features that are found in contemporary sphygmomanometers. The Janeway instrument had an extensible U-tube mercury manometer, it was portable, the armlet contained an inflatable bladder measuring 12 x 18 cm, and it was reasonably priced at US$14 [16].

William Dock has commented that *"the most remarkable fact about the Korotkoff sound is that it was discovered"* [16]. What is even more remarkable is that the sounds had been discovered some years before Korotkoff published his masterly paper. In 1901, Theodore Janeway, published a twenty page review of blood pressure measurement in the New York University Bulletin of the Medical Sciences in which he wrote: *"... that certain experiments in a number of cases concerning the pressure tone and murmur in the brachial, to be described later, show that the production of the tone always occurs at a lower pressure than the point in question (disappearance of secondary waves)"* [1]. He concluded the paper with another tantalising statement that undoubtedly indicates that he was well

1. Janeway T.C. Some observations on the estimation of blood pressure in man, with especial reference to the value of the results obtained with the newer sphygmomanometers. *New York Bull Med Sci* 1901; 105-126.

2. Janeway T.C. Diagnosis Significance of High Aterial Pressure. *Am J Med Sci* 1906; 131: 772-778.

3. Janeway T.C. The pathological physiology of chronic arterial hypertension and its treatment. *Trans Ass Am Physicians* 1906; 21:193-200.

4. Janeway T.C. The pathological physiology of chronic arterial hypertension and its treatment. *Am J Med Sci* 1907; 132:50-55.

5. Janeway T.C. A modification of the Riva-Rocci method of determining blood-pressure for use on the dog. *Proc Soc Exp Biol Med* 1909; 6:108-109.

6. Janeway T.C. The influence of the soft tissues of the arm on clinical blood-pressure determinations. *Arch Int Med* 1909; 3:474.

7. Janeway T.C. Note on Blood-pressure Changes Following Reduction of the Renal Arterial Circulation. *Proc Soc Exp Biol & Med* 1909; 6:109-111.

8. Janeway T.C. When should the general practitioner measure the blood pressure? *Albany M Ann* 1911; 32:159-168.

9. Janeway T.C. A study of the causes of death in one hundred patients with high blood pressure. *J Am Med Assn* 1912; 59:2106-2110.

10. Janeway T.C., Park E.A. The question of epinephrin in the circulation and its relation to blood pressure. *J Exp Med* 1912; 16: 541.

on the way to making a notable discovery: "*It is to be hoped that some more satisfactory method for estimating mean arterial pressure may yet be devised. I have been making some experiments on the tone and murmur produced in the brachial artery by known pressures, thinking that some information might thus be obtained. The results will be reported in a subsequent article together with a consideration of the value of our present methods from a clinical standpoint*" [1]. Unfortunately Janeway did not elaborate on this intriguing statement and he makes no mention of auscultatory phenomena in his extensive monograph written in 1904. Had he done so, we might speak of "Janeway sounds" but such is Korotkoff's succinct description that eponymous approbation cannot be challenged.

Janeway was clearly aware of the variability of blood pressure and he stressed the importance of making repeated observations of blood pressure [15]. In a series of remarkable clinical experiments he demonstrates graphically the striking response of blood pressure to stresses, such as surgery, tobacco and anxiety [15]. He was aware that the variable outcome in patients with hypertension was not related to the height of blood pressure alone but to the effect that raised blood pressure had on the target organs, particular the arterial circulation. "*I am confirmed in this opinion by certain individual cases in which extraordinary high pressures were tolerated for six years and more, while other patients with very moderate elevation of pressure died in a much shorter time. While, therefore, the medians of the living and the deceased groups do seem to show a certain unfavourable significance of blood-pressures above 200 mm, I consider the height of the blood-pressure a minor factor in determining the expectancy of life*" [13].

11. Janeway T.C. Nephritic Hypertension: Clinical and experimental studies. *Amer J Med Sci* 1913; 145:625-656.

12. Janeway T.C. A clinical study of hypertensive cardiovascular disease. *Trans Ass Am Physicians* 1913; 28: 333-386.

13. Janeway T.C. A clinical study of hypertensive cardiovascular disease. *Arch Int Med* 1913; 12:755-797.

14. Janeway T.C. Important contributions to clinical medicine during the past thirty years from the study of human blood pressure. *John Hopkins Hosp Bull* 1915; 26:341-350.

15. Janeway T.C. *The Clinical Study of Blood-Pressure.* D. Appleton & Co. New York and London. 1904.

16. O'Brien E., Fitzgerald D. The history of indirect blood pressure measurement. In: Blood Pressure Measurement. E. O'Brien and K. O'Malley Eds. *Handbook of hypertension.* W.H. Birkhager and J.L. Reid Eds. Elsevier. Amsterdam. 1991. pp. 1-54.

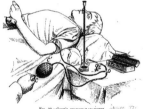

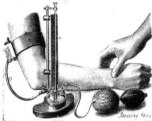

Two pages of Janeway's major work *The Clinical Study of Blood Pressure* (1904, D. Appleton & Co., New York and London.)

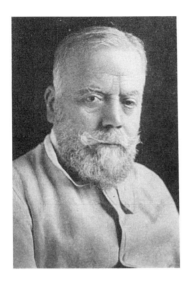

Henri Vaquez (1860-1936)

Henri Vaquez is a major figure in French medicine in general, and in the history of hypertension in particular. He was a student of Potain, to whom he owed his specialisation. He played an important role in popularising the measurement of blood pressure in man, and was a critic of Potain's sphygmomanometer. In collaboration with the manufacturer Galante, Vaquez produced his famous "sphygmotensiophone", based on Riva-Rocci's inflatable cuff principle and on Korotkoff's auscultatory method. The device was used by clinicians world-wide. Vaquez had doubts about the information derived simply by measuring the maximum and minimum blood pressures and so began working on the concept of "mean arterial pressure" and oscillometry.

His position as a consultant to a life insurance company made him acutely aware of the importance of high blood pressure as a risk factor. He was particularly interested in the role of the adrenals in hypertension and also in eclampsia. In therapeutics, his contribution to the action of nitrites in hypertension was noteworthy. A strong proponent of radiology, he developed many of its applications in cardiology and his Treatise on the radiology of the heart (Traité de radiologie du coeur) first published in 1921, ran to several editions. As a witness to the advent of electrocardiography, he also developed new concepts regarding cardiac rhythm disturbances.

Vaquez was a great communicator and author of many works. In 1908, he founded the journal Archives of the heart, vessels and blood (Archives du coeur, des vaisseaux et du sang) published by Baillère, which today remains one of the historical treasures of 20th century cardiology in France. It is noteworthy that when the journal was founded, haematology and cardiology were not separate entities. Vaquez worked with Malassez at the Collège de France and described polycythaemia vera, a condition which today bears his name.

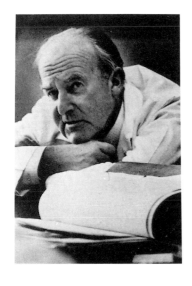

George Pickering (Sir) (1904-1980)

The name of Sir George Pickering is closely linked to the recent history of hypertension. He was a staunch defender of the "Fallacy of the dividing line" between normal and pathological blood pressure. He showed that blood pressure was continuously distributed (contrary to Platt's belief of a bimodal distribution) and that therefore hypertension could not be defined other than by arbitrary numbers.

In the 1930s, George Pickering (with Prinzmetal) "rediscovered" renin which had been described 30 years before by Tigerstedt and Bergman, and he perceived that the renin-angiotensin system served as a long-term regulator of blood pressure.

In the 1950s, he conceived and performed a series of technically difficult experiments to show that an increase in arterial pressure could be induced and maintained by intravenous infusion of renin.

From 1939 to 1956, George Pickering was department head at St. mary's Hospital, where he did his major work on hypertension. It was with the support and encouragement of Pickering that Peart, who had worked in Pickering's department at St. Mary's hospital, isolated angiotensin, then determined its amino-acid sequence in collaboration with Elliot at Mill Hill.

Pickering went on to pioneer continous blood pressure recording in collaboration with colleagues in Oxford, thus opening up what continues to be a very fruitful area of physiological and clinical investigation.

The author of a major textbook on hypertension, Pickering's gift for public speaking, his talent for writing and his fearless, but just criticisms made him a an impotant and influential figure in the development of the field of hypertension.

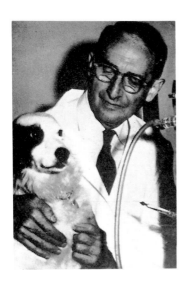

Harry Goldblatt

Harry Goldblatt was one of the few researchers who, in the early 1930s, was devoting most of his time to laboratory work on hypertension. In 1934, he achieved the first reproducible animal model of hypertension by clamping the renal arteries of dogs. He thereby clarified the numerous theories on the relationship between renal alterations and elevated blood pressure. His landmark publication appeared in the *Journal of Experimental Medicine*...after being rejected by the *American Heart Journal.*

Irvin Page

Irvin Page's career coincides with the recent history of hypertension. In 1940 Page's group in Cleveland co-discovered angiotensin (which they called angiotonin). Page published his memoirs under the title *Hypertension Research — a memoir 1920-1960* (1988, Pergamon Press, N.Y.).

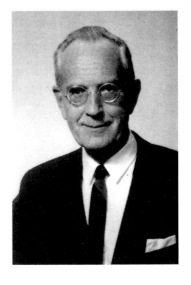

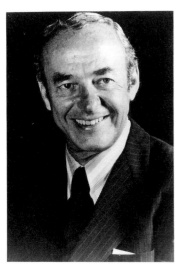

Edward Freis

Edward Freis spent most of his career at the Veterans Administration Hospital in Washington DC and was Professor of medicine at Georgetown University Medical Centre. He introduced the use of thiazide diuretics in the treatment of hypertension. He was instrumental in demonstrating the clinical activity of antihypertensive agents and their efficacy in reducing cardiovascular mortality in hypertensive patients. He received the Lasker prize for his work in 1971.

INDEX OF NAMES

Achard 117
Ackerknecht 68
Addison 111
Adson 121
Ahlquist 128
Alexander 129
Allbutt 60, 167
Allen 119, 135, 138
Ambard 93, 117, 118, 119
Annest 182
Arsonval (d') 106, 107, 108
Aubertin 82
Auclair 114
Auenbrugger 172
Axelrad 76
Ayman 24, 26, 168, 181
Bakhle 130
Banting 73
Barger 127
Barnad 202
Basch 10, 13, 20, 26, 59, 63, 68, 102
Baxter 114
Beaujard 93, 117, 118, 119
Bergmann 73, 75
Bergognié 110
Bernard 60, 64, 68, 72, 107, 133, 134, 142
Best 73
Bevan 23, 30
Beyer 98
Bichat 38, 67
Bickford 23
Black 99, 128
Blackburn 148
Bordet 173
Boulitte 20
Brand 34
Braun-Mendez 76
Brest 96
Bright 743, 44, 64, 67, 68, 69, 70, 71, 72, 102,
    167, 172, 178
Broca 110
Broussais 102
Brown-Séquard 72, 73, 107
Brucer 138, 139
Brush 45
Buffon 32
Buhler 132
Canguilhem 133
Cannon 127, 128
Casale 178
Cash 75

Céline 155
Challamel 107, 108
Clark 127
Cohn 101
Collip 73
Conn 59, 64, 65, 77, 78, 79, 87, 88, 90
Corvisart 38, 67, 172, 173
Corvol 186
Cottard 91
Cottenot 111, 112
Cournot 34, 49
Craig 121
Cushing 28, 29, 199
Cushman 130
Dagonet 10, 101
Dale 127, 128
Davis 32, 77
Dawber 52
Deadborn 24
Delherm 110
Deparcieux 32
Desplats 113
Devereux 178
Dieulafoy 181
Dock 202
Dominguez 75
Donzelot 135, 174
Dooren 113
Doumer 82
Dumas 63, 111, 113
Dustan 97, 126
Dutch 176
Duvillard 32
Einthoven 176
Elliot 76, 205
Engel 23, 83
Engelman 83, 84
Erdös 130
Fabre 149
Fagot-Largeault 54, 58
Fahr 75, 94
Faivre 10
Farr 50
Faught 46
Federov 200
Ferreira 130
Ferrié 110
Ferry 27
Fischer 35, 45, 46, 47, 54
Fishberg 118
Flaubert 150

Fleckenstein 131
Fontaine 89
Forlanini 199
Foucault 49
Fränkel 79, 80
Freis 123, 124, 127, 206
Freud 106
Frost 47
Furberg 132
Gaddum 127
Gaertner 23, 107, 108
Galante 204
Gallavardin 24, 26, 27, 63, 64, 136, 138, 189
Genest 77
Gernier 9
Gilbert 110
Giraud 64
Godfraind 131
Goldblatt 74, 75, 76, 79, 121, 130, 206
Goormaghtigh 77
Gordon 74
Graunt 32, 36
Grawitz 74
Grmek 19
Gross 77
Guazzi 132
Gull 67, 69, 72
Hales 9, 19, 59, 133
Halphen 114
Hamet 114, 117
Hamilton 139
Hansson 129
Haour 24
Hartman 75
Hartroft 77
Harvey 133, 171
Heitz 174
Helmcke 178
Hérisson 9
Hill 202
Hines 101
Hinman 23
Hippocrates 11, 27, 32, 134, 145
Honour 23
Houghton 118
Howell 45
Huchard 63, 64, 102, 117, 118
Hunter 47
Illich 180
Israel 74
Jaboulay 121

Janeway 24, 26, 35, 45, 75, 159, 173, 202, 203
Jeannel 40
Jeunemaître 186
Kannel 51, 175
Kaplan 162
Katzenstein 75
Keith 94, 95, 97
Kempner 118, 121
Koch 58, 134
Korotkoff 14, 20, 200, 201, 202, 203
Krayer 101
Labbé 79, 80, 81, 82, 83, 84
Lacroix 156
Laënnec 10, 38, 67, 173
Laguerrière 110
Lahy 9
Laignel-Lavastine 82
Lander 186
Langeron 113
Langley 127
Laplace 32, 34
Laragh 77
Lathrop 186
Laubry 14, 63, 114, 159, 176
Le Pen 162
Leconte 174
Lemmer 23
Lemoine 108
Leriche 63, 68, 121, 142
Levy 89
Lewinski 74
Lian 51, 150, 151
Liddle 184
Lifton 184
Loéper 31, 48
Louis 34, 50, 102
Ludwig 9, 71
Luetscher 76
Lyons 96
Mac Leod 73
Mackenzie 47, 51, 58
Mahomed 60
Malassez 204
Marey 10, 19, 28, 41, 102, 107
Maseri 132
Mayo 79, 81, 82, 83, 84
Melot 113
Ménard 164
Millian 13, 14
Moran 128
Morgagni 43, 178

Moritz 42, 43
Mosso 23
Moutier 106, 107, 108, 110
Mulon 111
Murray 73 Ng 130
O'Brien 20, 28
Oliver 80
Ondetti 130
Pachon 20, 80, 112
Page 76, 97, 114, 126, 139, 206
Pahor 132
Paillard 20
Pasteur 58
Peart 76, 205
Pedersen 75
Peet 94, 121, 122, 123
Pellissier 47, 176
Perera 98, 139
Perkins 128
Pick 82
Pickering 57, 64, 123, 135, 139, 143, 182, 205
Pincoffs 79, 82, 83, 84
Pinell 51
Piquemal 34, 50
Platt 57, 139, 182, 205
Poiseuille 9, 20, 133
Potain 13, 16, 24, 26, 27, 59, 63, 68, 102, 107, 118, 155, 173, 204
Pratt 168
Price 32
Prichard 129
Prineas 148
Proust 91
Psaty 132
Radiguet 106
Rapp 185
Raynaud 51, 114
Reaven 150
Richet 114
Riesman 54, 111
Riva-Rocci 13, 16, 20, 23, 25, 26, 107, 155, 199, 202, 204
Robin 102
Robinson 135, 138, 139
Roger 47
Röntgen 111, 173
Rosenbleuth 127, 128
Rosenbloom 181
Roth 83
Rousseau 145
Rowntree 121

Ruyter 77
Schild 127
Scholtz 45, 47, 48
Schwartz 54
Schwyzer 76
Sénac 172
Shanks 128
Shaw 74
Sheps 84
Simpson 76, 88
Skeggs 76, 130
Smirk 185
Smithwick 94, 121, 122, 123
Snavely 80
Sokolow 23, 28, 176
Spengler 14
Starling 172
Stévenin 47, 146
Stolz 80
Stott 23
Sulser 77
Susser 51
Sutton 72, 83
Taylor 114
Tesla 106
Tigerstedt 73, 75
Tinel 82
Totti 31
Traube 71, 72, 75, 102
Trousseau 87, 90
Valéry 167
Valsalva 20
Vane 130
Vaquez 412, 14, 47, 64, 71, 82, 108, 112, 140, 173, 176, 204
Vaschide 9
Verdin 107
Vierodt 10
Vleminckx 37
Volhard 94
Vulpian 80
Wagener 94, 95, 97
White 51
Widal 91, 108, 117
Wilkins 123
Williams 183
Woley 46
Wood 75
Yanovski 201
Zacharias 129
Zimmern 111